THE **KARMA** HANDBOOK

REINCARNATION AND HEALING

TRUTZ HARDO

JAICO PUBLISHING HOUSE

Ahmedabad Bangalore Chennai
Delhi Hyderabad Kolkata Mumbai

Published by Jaico Publishing House
A-2 Jash Chambers, 7-A Sir Phirozshah Mehta Road
Fort, Mumbai - 400 001
jaicopub@jaicobooks.com
www.jaicobooks.com

Published in arrangement with
Verlag "Die Silberschnur" GmbH
Steinstraße 1
D-56593 Güllesheim
Germany

To be sold only in India, Bangladesh, Bhutan,
Pakistan, Nepal, Sri Lanka and the Maldives.

THE KARMA HANDBOOK
ISBN 978-81-8495-908-6

First Jaico Impression: 2016

Printed by
Repro India Limited, Mumbai

Contents

Introduction

Whoever makes visible the complex paths of karma does a service to mankind.

(H.P.Blavatsky)

The concept of karma or karman comes from Sanskrit, originally meaning deed, doing, acting, work, action. Everything is thus named which results from doing. This karma is connected with a law according to which everything I do – as well as everything that I think and say – has its consequences. If I do good things, good things will be done to me; if I do evil things, they will also be my lot. These are the actions of my soul. But because my soul lives a number of consecutive lives as a human being, this law is not necessarily enforced in my present life, but usually in a later life, whether this is the immediately consecutive or a later one. Based on cause and effect, e.g. action and reaction, it works just as the (better known) physical law of "cause and effect" does – for example as seen in the "law of gravity": the higher the object the more destruction it causes upon falling.

What led me to write this book was the wish to inform mankind of the fundamental and axiomatic validity of the law of karma. It is just as fundamentally – i.e. indisputably – and axiomatically true as e.g. the law of gravity! From the unnecessary ignorance and resulting inattention of the majority of mankind toward this law a great amount of unnecessary suffering also occurs – suffering for the individual as well as for the human race as a whole!

But I do not want to set before the reader another one of those usual repetitious books on karma of which there are probably hundreds. Rather I would like to present a totally new book on the realities of karma. Namely, I want to describe here the often quite new concepts evolving from my daily occupation as a regression therapist.

In the first part of the book I introduce the reader to Indian thought on karma in general. The third part is the main part, in which I would like to show the effects of the law of karma by demonstrating them on thirty-one cases of Regression Therapy. The second part gives the reader a short introduction to Regression Therapy, helping him or her to understand the third part better.

Almost ninety percent of all humans believe in an at least partial supernatural intervention into the private and public fate of mankind. Of these about half believe in repeated life on earth, i.e. in reincarnation. And of these latter most see reincarnation as connected with the effects produced by the law of karma. But up to now there was still no "scientific proof" for these two fundamental laws of life.

With his monumental work *Reincarnation and Biology* (1997), Ian Stevenson, professor at the University of Virginia in Charlottesville, U.S.A., has achieved no less a feat than demonstrating reincarnation conclusively to be a fact. And I would like to be just as bold in undertaking with the present book the attempt to prove conclusively the law of karma to be a fact![1]

---

1. The reader can find his most important publications listed in the Bibliography under *Proofs for Reincarnation*, above all his more then 2200 pages book *Reincarnation and Biology* which he summarized for "the man of the road" in his shorter book *Where Reincarnation and Biology Intersect*. But he has written those books in a scientific language, which may not be so palatable to the common reader. For this reason I have written two books (*Rebirth – The evidence* and *Children who have lived before*) which not only present some of the most important of Stevenson's documentations in a more readable style but also include proofs and background material on reincarnation from numerous other sources.

What gives me the courage to make such a statement? For many years I have been active as a regression therapist in Germany and abroad, training also others in Regression Therapy. Not only I personally, but probably all regression therapists worldwide, have repeatedly discovered – along with the root causes for their clients' symptoms – conclusive evidence for the validity of the law of karma.

Let us take a look at the treatment, for example, in our office of a woman with chronic constant coughing. After leading her to the cause of her disease and guiding her to the point where she can see herself at the moment in the Middle Ages when she is being burned as a witch, we then delve further into why she had to suffer this fate. We will inevitably find an earlier life in which she was an agent in causing the same or a similar fate, helping directly or indirectly to destroy someone else by burning. This then is the real cause of her present situation.

And regression therapists could prove in hundreds of thousands of such cases that this law – „What ye have done to others, so shall ye suffer thyself" – is constantly and definitely manifesting itself. This cannot be only by chance. If Carl Gustav Jung was still unsatisfied as a scientist with the firm belief in the reality of reincarnation and karma by Indian philosophers – in his opinion empirical proof then being lacking[2] – we can now say, as regression therapists confronted daily with the effects of this law, that even from the empirical standpoint it has finally to be accepted as irrefutable. Not only the fact that our clients' symptoms unfold under its magical sway allows us to speak with such certainty of the validity of the

2. Hanson, p. 131

karmic law. There is also the fact that understanding the law itself allows them to overcome its aftereffects and often even to experience an immediate release from its symptoms!

Such successes in healing are in my opinion the surest and most valid proof for the reality of the karmic law. While reading the third part of this book the reader will be astounded how overwhelming these successes are – successes of which contemporary medicine and psychotherapy can only dream. For the same reason they also will not be able to ignore this form of therapy in the long run.

Cooperation between (psycho-)medical practitioners and regression therapists will necessarily evolve. These successes in the area of somatic, psychosomatic and psychic treatment will be passed by word-of-mouth to sufferers in the respective areas. A huge army of doctors and therapists with training in Regression Therapy will then be necessary in order to handle the great demand. Other regression therapists will possibly demonstrate (as I have done) at professional congresses or in TV the wonders of Regression Therapy, so that everyone should soon be convinced of the rapid effect of this therapy form. But above all the insurance companies will be willing to pay for the training of regression therapists, as they will soon notice how many million dollars can be saved by this treatment, which is generally the quickest and most effective method. Furthermore, Regression Therapy has the spiritual result that even the client's soul can experience a healing effect, if it, by accepting the karmic law, no longer deviates from the path of righteousness and love (dharma). But Regression Therapy should not be a privilege reserved only for the ill and suffering – everyone can greatly profit from insight into his/her past actions.

This book should obviously not only be of interest to the general reader, but also to all those persons concerned with healing .They should be especially open to and interested in these new treatment methods. Therefore the reader is encouraged to make such persons aware of this book or possibly even to present it to them as a gift of a very special kind.

The fourth part is of no less importance than the third. In many respects karma will be shown here in a completely new light and within a new framework, namely on the basis of the insights gained from Regression Therapy. For instance, there is an important fact that has hardly received any consideration throughout the whole previous history of karma research and philosophy: We ourselves – in the period of "afterlife" before beginning a new life – have determined the amount and type of "karmic baggage" to be carried in our coming life. This we have done on the basis of the karmic material still to be dissolved and with the help of the advisors in the beyond who aided us in planning our life to come. So we have taken upon ourselves everything we encounter in life and that even the worst karmic experiences in every life are previously chosen – or at least accepted – by us previous to entering upon this new life. This can be certified to by all those regression therapists who take their clients back to the time before their entry into a new life on earth.

In America there is an excellent researcher on this topic who, with the help of his clients, has given us in recent years some completely new revelations on this area of "the beyond", including the preparations made for karmic re-entry. He is Dr. Michael Newton, and his name will probably soon be just as well-known in research on the karma and the beyond as that of Professor Ian Stevenson in the area of reincarnation. Whatever truths have revealed themselves through modern research into reincarnation have been due to the memories stemming from the subconscious of thousands of clients. And if thousands - soon hundreds of thousands – of clients repeat the same basic – and often very logical – facts, there will be common denominators that can stand up to critical scientific testing. On the basis of this research we can now maintain that knowledge of the basic truths of existence and fundamental self-knowledge about one's own existence is hidden in the subconscious of every individual person. When these basic truths are uncovered, they may be viewed or explained differently in detail, revealing many common principles never consciously available to normal persons outside of trance.

My own experiences in reincarnation duplicate those experiences of the beyond described by Dr. Newton. In addition I have been able to discover as an empirical fact that we ourselves have by our own higher consciousness set up our own basic karmic "burden" because we wanted for very special reasons to experience personally the different forms of suffering.

In the forth part of this book I have collected as well the different previously known forms of karma, supplemented them by various new forms arising through our experiences with Regression Therapy, and catalogued them in 23 different types. No one who aims to do research on karma in the future would be advised to ignore this data. As human beings we need no longer remain "in the dark" about reincarnation and karma. Researchers have now delved by hypnotism and trance into the previously little-known secret vaults of mankind, shedding the light of the subconscious on the treasures hidden there. These newly discovered treasures should now eliminate the need for speculating on possible "hidden lodes" (as earlier belief-systems and researchers have done), because such speculations have now largely become superfluous. Of course, there will be even more treasures to discover, and certainly there will also be some major surprises in store for us. The present book aims to reveal some of these discoveries, and I wish the reader great pleasure in perusing them!

Part One

India as the birthplace of the karmic concept

From the concept of reincarnation to the first karma concept

The world will only be cured of its ills when knowledge of karma and reincarnation has spread throughout the whole world. Without this knowledge there is no cure, no truth, no honesty, no peace and no Golden Age.

(Sai Baba)

The complete history of karmic thought in human history has not been written yet and is still waiting to find proper consideration in an extensive book. However, the following brief treatment may serve the uninitiated reader as an introduction. It is based on karmic thought in India.

India is generally known as the birthplace of the karmic concept. Indians maintain this claim with pride, because they see this great religious and philosophical contribution to the study of truth as an integral part of their heritage. Therefore they deny categorically all theories that would diminish this claim.

The oldest texts on religious concepts in India were compiled in the *Vedas* – based on the foregoing oral or written tradition before the 6th century B.C. and presenting very differing standpoints. On the one hand there is mention of a final judge *Yama* (similar to Hades in the ancient Greek tradition), who allots out punishment to souls after death. Here there is the concept of eternal hellish punishment as well as that of eternal enjoyment in heavenly spheres. On the other hand there is already mention of reincarnation or transformation of humans into animal bodies or into those of other humans, mostly relatives, though at other places reincarnation seems to be completely denied and death is seen as a ruthless destroyer.

In other scriptures there is mention of a person's liberation from eternal birth and death if he/she has regularly and properly carried out the prescribed ritualistic offering ceremonies. (Here the desire of the priestly castes to maintain their prerogatives is evident.) In another scripture, meat-eating persons are threatened with being devoured themselves in the afterlife. In general, we can say that retribution is seen here – in a similar way to that later in Christianity – as taking place after the end of life in an "afterlife" area, i.e. "beyond" the worldly sphere.

In the *Chandogya Upanishad* the law of karma is stated for the first time as retribution causality in connection with reincarnation. According to this script everyone carrying out a pious life will be reincarnated into one of the higher castes: priests, warriors or tradesmen, while those with impious lives are fated to take birth as dogs, swine or humans without a caste.

However, the passages in this *Upanishad* raise the question (according to the researcher Halbfass)[3] of possibly having been interpolated into the scriptures at a later time, because they pop up suddenly and without any apparent reason in the text. Such interpolations were, as we know from Christian Biblical research, commonly used to introduce the opinions of later generations into the older texts while copying them, thus disguising them in the form of authentic original thoughts. So this formulation of the karmic concept seems relatively recent, probably not having been introduced

3. Halbfass, p. 52. In this short history of the concept of karma, I base my discussion of the ancient Indian concept of karma largely on the elaborations in this book, which includes a good up-to-date overview of present Indian scholarship in this field.

before the 4th Century B.C. Just as improbable is the age of the *Brihad-Aranyaka-Upanishad* alleged by religious Indians. Here the karmic law is formulated very clearly, without however mentioning its effect in attaining a higher caste. And one is supposed to be re-born in the next life according to the acts of his present life: Whoever carries out good acts will be born as a good person. "Whoever carries out evil acts will have an evil birth. One becomes holy by doing holy works, evil by evil works."[4]

In the *Brihad-Aranyaka-Upanishad* there is for the first time mention of freedom from evil desires as being the qualification for liberation from birth and death. And in this text the concept karma – in the sense that good actions bring about repeated auspicious earthly lives, bad actions inauspicious ones – also occurs for the first time[5]. But, as Halbfass points out, nowhere in the *Vedas* is there an example of the classic double-edged karmic axiom: No morally relevant acts without retribution [i.e. punishment or reward]. No positive or negative experiences without karmic causes.[6]

It was not until as late as the great epos *Mahabarata*, approximately 400 B.C. that this axiom turned up within Hinduism. In this most extensive epic of world literature we find unmistakable statements of the karmic law: "The deed follows the doer like his shadow" or "All living beings experience the results of their actions" or "What is sowed will also be harvested" or "Good and bad karma never disappears." And in the 12th book the God *Kala* explains that he himself – as the God of Time – has no personal

4. Zander, p. 28
5. Halbfass, p. 55f.
6. Halbfass, p. 62.

power and that he himself is subject to karmic law. [7]

The "jewel" of the *Mahabarata* is however the *Bhagavad-gita*, rating as the "New Testament" of Hindu *Vishnuism*. Here reincarnation is mentioned frequently while referring to the fact that the soul eternally lives in various bodies. The unequivocal karmic law, namely that goodness leads to higher knowledge, while passion incurs renewed reincarnation, is also explained there:

If good things grow in man, he reaches after death
Those blameless realms of highest wisdom.
In passion dying, he returns amongst the doers,
But if in darkness, he's born from deluded womb anew.
The fruit of righteous deed is good existence pure,
Passion has to suffer, but ignorance is darkness' fruit.
From goodness wisdom, from passion careless desire,
Deluded sense - unknowing - from the darkness stems.
Those rich in goodness shall climb aloft.[8]

The *Vedas* and the early *Upanishads* - in contrast to the later *Upanishads* - say nothing about karma, while the *Bhagavad-gita* was probably not written before the 3rd Century B.C. This leads to the conjecture that Jainism or Buddhism or another source may have influenced this great Hindu-Bible in its interpretation of the karmic law. It supports also the assumption that the rapid expansion of Buddhism and Jainism with their reincarnation teachings had reached the point where the Brahmans, who felt themselves to be the protectors of the Vedas and of Hinduism, made the effort to introduce this concept of reincarnation and

7. Bhagavadgita, Song 2, Couplet 30, also Song 4, Couplet 5, Song 7, Couplet 19, Song 8, Couplet 15f. etc.
8. Bhagavadgita, Song 14, Couplet 14ff.

karma into their scriptures.[9] Many researchers believe therefore that the concept of reincarnation may have been part of a tribal religion existing before the Aryanisation of India, perhaps infusing itself later at some time into the older and newer religious traditions. Or do these influences stem from somewhere else?

But even before this gigantic work was written and compiled there were in India two great religious movements that had added so to speak the "walls" to the karmic "foundation" of the *Upanishads*. These movements, each founded by a great visionary, have already been mentioned here: Jainism and Buddhism.

The concept of karma in Jainism

The founder of Jainism, *Vardhamana Mahavira*, was an older contemporary of Buddha. Both of them lived allegedly between 580 and 480 B.C., but there are also researchers who set that one hundred years later. More fable than fact has been related about their lives. Each of them founded an oral tradition whose later compilers obviously added many ideas of their own, intending to extend, deepen or just modify the original teachings in a way not always in complete agreement with the original.

The true founding scripture of Jainism – that later split into two branches: the *Digambaras* and the *Svetambaras* - is called the *Tattvarthasutra* or *Tattvarthadhigamasutra* and was only compiled about 700 years after the death of its founder by a man named *Umasvati*. Thus it is hard to say with certainty what *Mahavira* himself actually developed in the way of new karmic concepts. According to tradition at least,

9. Zander, p. 41

he developed astounding new approaches that may have been a decisive influence on the development of both Buddhism and Hinduism. Of course, all of these three great movements – Hinduism, Buddhism and Jainism – have influenced each other mutually.

According to Jainism every soul stems from a non-material world but has become entangled in the material world as we know it. Now the soul must struggle to escape from his entanglement in this material world. And what prevents the soul from escaping, i.e. from final liberation from the wheel of birth and rebirth, is karma (in Pali also known as *kamma*).

Karma or *kamma* binds the soul, which is only able to free itself from samsara, the wheel of worldly activity (the wheel of eternal birth and rebirth) on the basis of decisive knowledge, by giving up all material wishes and desires and by becoming free of sexual desires and of all impurities of the soul, such as anger, vanity, pride, desire, jealousy, dishonesty etc. It must consciously practice *ahimsa*, i.e. freedom from aggression by eating no meat, killing no living beings, not even the tiniest creature, to ultimately attain freedom from all material attachments. This, of course, requires great willpower.

I have myself lived with the monks of the *Svetambara* sect, walking with them many kilometers by foot. I have also translated the works of their leader, His Holiness *Asare Sri Tulsi*, from English into German.

According to him, every impure thought, word or action

10. Shri Nemichandra S. Chakravarti's book lists all the different ideas of the Jains about karma. It is also interesting to note the list of times - precise down to the minute - related to different karmic reactions (p. 25).

solidifies attachment to the material world and makes it impossible to attain in this life liberation from the wheel of birth and rebirth. In order to train willpower and to free oneself from all possible attractions there are many exercises, among which the practice of fasting for weeks or even for one or two months is the most popular.

According to the belief of the Jains, the earthly universe is composed of tiny material karma particles that we allow by our material thoughts to get into our souls. Impure thoughts, above all, open wide the gates through which these particles can flow into our souls. The key is then to allow no further particles into our soul, or, if they do somehow enter, to remove them again. Because these particles, if still attached to our souls at death, cause us to immediately return to a material body, without even having the possibility of an enjoyable pause in the "the beyond" state between material lives.

The vibrations allowing entrance of such material particles into our bodies are of two types: those that are caused by passions coming from thoughts, words or deeds in our bodies and those that gain entrance without our transmitting such thoughts or passions. Though "only" the first group causes karma, the mass of karma composed of such karma particles can still easily cover our knowledge of the truth, for which reason so many people lack the desire to know the truth. They also open our senses for earthly desires, disturbing our energy and even reducing our lifespan.

There is hindering karma, destructive, non-destructive, confusing karma and many other kinds of karma resulting from the concentration of karma particles that occupy the soul and the body. The Jainist teachings on karma, which is the central element of their belief, are extraordinarily complicated, being separated into many different parts. There are hundreds of karmic causes that have been catalogued. One hundred and forty-eight types of karma have been discovered up to now. Even 93 kinds of karmic results and the duration of the effects of certain covering karma particles and their number have been established.

The greater part of this labyrinth of karmic complications can be recited by memory by Jain monks, who make five vows before entering a monastery: ahimsa (non-violence), honesty (no lies), no taking of others' property (stealing), sexual renunciation and finally no desire for material possessions. Therefore they have no temples, no land and property, no houses, no possessions for themselves besides the necessities of life that they carry with themselves. To the latter belong also their extensive libraries written with microscopically small letters on palm leaves. On each palm leaf about 50 normal pages can be written. Among the many virtues that they are supposed to practice in order to remove the karma particles from the body, neutralize them or protect against them: friendliness to all, empathy, equanimity and joyful sensitivity without envy.

The meaning of karma in Buddhism

Siddharta Gautama, later known as Buddha, lived first like *Mahavira* in renunciation, before he discovered his "middle way" between worldly renunciation and attachment to the world. After attaining enlightenment, he spent more than 40 years as a wandering preacher in order to spread his teachings, which were only recorded in writing three to four centuries later. Various versions with differing commentaries have evolved, leading to the development of different schools of thought. For instance, the questions were variously discussed of the number of times Buddha had incarnated and/or how many lives he had actually been able to remember, if he had ever taken an animal body, that of a woman etc.

The first night of his enlightenment he is supposed – according to the *Theravada* school – to have remembered innumerable previous lives. Looking further back, he was supposed to have remembered different world destructions and rebuilding periods. In the second night he recognized what happens to human beings after death, i.e. the karmic path they acquire according to their thoughts and deeds. Those who have acted badly in thought, word and deed go to hell because of this negative karma. On the other hand those who have produced good karma go to heaven.

The karmic concept is not yet connected with reincarnation here, although these souls are expected at some time to incarnate again. In the third night the three basic evils were revealed to – the now enlightened – Buddha and how they can be overcome and destroyed. The first evil is sensory desire, the second ambition and the third ignorance. When the human being overcomes these evils, he is released from the chain of repetitive lives on earth, and Buddha could say of himself at that point: "I will never return to this world."

In other scriptures – probably compiled and interpolated by disciples of the disciples of his own disciples – he connected karma with reincarnation.[11] For him suffering is

---

11. Zander (p. 41) confirms that in the body of works believed to contain Buddha's original teachings reincarnation actually plays only a minor role. Most of the statements on this subject seem to have been added by later disciples, who placed more emphasis on it.

connected with life, and renewed lives of suffering on earth happen through acquired karma. In order to free oneself from this suffering and the contingent karma, he recommends an eight-fold path: right beliefs, right decisions, right words, right deeds, right life, right striving, right thinking, right meditating.[12] In a conversation with a young Brahmin, *Subha,* Buddha explains the karmic law explicitly: There is on the basis of one's deeds karma that comes to fruition in the present life and other karma that only comes to fruition in one's next life on earth. That means that we ourselves cause on the basis of our previous and present activities the nature of our coming existences on earth.

This is the first time that karma is connected by him with renewed life, i.e. with reincarnation. To King *Malika Buddha* says that people become ugly or receive outer blemishes because they carried out unfriendly activities in earlier lives. *Theravada Buddhism* distinguishes now also good karma (*kusala*) from bad (*akusala*) karma. It depends always on the intention connected to one's thoughts, speech or works. In this way the extent of fault and faultlessness is measured according to the intention, i.e. the motivation of the deed.

Representatives of *Sarvastivada Buddhism* also add to this: lack of sorrow and remorse in measuring karmic responsibility. Thus even through neutrality can one obtain negative karmic reactions. In Buddhism a soul can also become an ugly person or a pauper in his next life, but – differently than in Hinduism – one can never revert to the animal state.

The human being is also fully responsible for his destiny because this arises out of his previous actions, whether from

12. Friedli, p. 78

this or an earlier life. One's own personal free decision determines one's destiny, allowing one also to free oneself from the constrictions of karma by carrying out proper action. Proper action is, however, based on knowledge and dependent on one's own judgment. With proper use of these faculties one can free oneself from the cycle of birth and rebirth.

And - as in Jainism – the methods of attaining this goal are clearly stated in the scriptures: By knowledge one knows that passion keeps the wheel of rebirth moving. If one acts on this knowledge to stop passion, then automatically all impulses of the will are reduced. Thus no new karma occurs, helping to prepare one for liberation in nirvana - that indescribable state of unrestricted bliss, free of desires and ego.

At this point we could actually close our description of the Buddhist karma concept, based on cause and effect, if there were not also scriptures claiming Buddha as their source in which the existence of a transmigrating soul is denied. The problem with this is that if the soul does not exist in reality then it can also never be reborn. This "pseudo-soul" would thus be eliminated by definition or at least be destroyed at death, being only a construction of the life-energy and the ego.

This problem has been the source of extended religious and philosophical controversy, as well as of numerous sectarian divisions. Of course such hair-splitting has always only confused the masses of everyday believers. For them simpler formulas of soul transmigration and karmic retribution with the possibility of a final liberation in nirvana have been proclaimed.

The widely varying commentaries of subsequent centuries

compiled different ways how karma could be caused. To sum them up we can say: Five basic moral rules allow not only monks, but also all believers to avoid karma: avoiding aggression, stealing, lies, sexual excess and alcoholic intoxication. For many Buddhists vegetarianism is also an anti-karma commandment, while others – e.g. the Dalai Lama - can occasionally eat meat without causing karmic reactions.

As with the Jains, the main causes of karmic complications are the passions: desire, hate, illusion (also including denial of the "truth"), killing, adultery, malice. There is a list of the "ten coverings": darkness, doubt, shamelessness etc., and also one of disturbances causing karmic reactions.

On the way to truth, i.e. the way to liberation from karmic entanglement and having to undergo repeated lives on earth, three drives must be overcome, namely sexuality, ambition and ignorance. If we finally overcome these passions, further instructions show us, for example, the "seven steps to oneness", leading us with certainty out of the eternal wheel of rebirth and allowing us to attain oneness with the final object of desire: nirvana.

Various streams within Buddhism may also accept intermediary existences in the beyond, before renewed incarnation takes place on earth. The classical representative of the Sarvastivada movement, *Vasubandhu*, gives an exact description of what happens after death. There the soul forms a ghost-body, the *gandharva*, which exists in the period between two earth lives in the beyond, guiding at the end of this period the soul to its place of rebirth in accordance with its previously caused karma. It can even be present at the time of copulation, viewing its prospective parents while they produce its own body-to-be. If it is to incarnate as a male, it can then feel hate for its future father and attraction for its mother. Or else it can feel, as a female, attraction for its future father and hate for its mother. Sigmund Freud would have applauded such a forerunner to his own Oedipal theories.

Mahayana Buddhism, among which also Tibetan Buddhism is counted, believes that Buddha renounced returning to nirvana because of his love for human beings, wanting to help them in their suffering and ignorance. Therefore he is still incarnating in the more advanced lamas, e.g. the Dalai Lama, helping them by his accumulated good karma and his consequent goodness, love and knowledge to move toward liberation.

Structures of Indian karma models

Karma is both action and the consequence of that action; it is cause and effect simultaneously.

(Deepak Chopra)

In Hinduism, just as in Jainism and in Buddhism, the different descriptions in the existing scriptures, e.g. the *Vedas*, the *Upanishads*, the great epic works *Ramayana* and *Mahabharata*, as well as the many *sutras*, *puranas* and other scriptures including extended reproductions and commentaries, have led to very different streams and sub-streams.

Today six traditional Hindu systems are counted, namely the *Vaisesika*, *Nyaya*, *Samkhya*, *Yoga*, *Mimasa* and *Vedanta*. They have all occupied themselves with rebirth and karma, basing their respective theoretical systems on their opinions about these two concepts. These two concepts are even the hinges on which their religious and philosophical systems turn, including such questions as that of how to free oneself from *samsara* (the eternal wheel) through *dharma* (the pure path of morality).

To offer the reader an example of these many considerations I will discuss in the following several concepts of *Vyasa* which are also of interest for our further discussion of this topic:

Vyasa, who is known as a commentator of the *sutras* of *Patanjali* living in the fifth century A.D., distinguishes between

– actions arising from instinct and inborn behavioral tendencies as well as passions stemming from the drive for existence and self-protection, which exist automatically in all living beings as predispositions (*samskara*), and
– those carried out intentionally by thinking beings.

The first group is described as being largely free of karma. The latter group, described as actually responsible for causing karma, is again divided into two categories:

– major offenses such as stealing, lying, adultery, murder, fraud and
– minor offenses such as carelessness, lack of empathy or small misdeeds.

The total amount of karmic ballast accumulating from all these offenses directly forms the coordinates for the conditions determining one's next life. Though predispositions directed by instinct and the like are found in all life, they are found in a gradually diminishing degree in higher and higher levels of conscious life, being replaced more and more by conscious modes of choice. And the total amount of offenses consciously carried out in one life is directly responsible for the weight of karmic reactions in the following life. In other words: the greater the karmic ballast, the more difficult the following life. We therefore punish ourselves by encumbering ourselves with heavy karmic ballast, which manifests itself in the following life as difficulties causing suffering.

In other scriptures the distinction is made between "black (very bad) karma", "white (very good) karma" and "black and white (mixed) karma". If one has at present a very nice life, the previous life must have been filled with white karma. This is in contrast to a life where one as a result of black karma finds oneself among the despised classes of society (persons without caste) or afflicted with a terrible illness. But most people carry both white and black karma and have therefore a mixed bag of suffering and joy.

The most famous Indian philosopher and advocate of the *Vedanta* system is *Shankara*, who lived around 700 A.D. He was mostly concerned with self-knowledge as a means to transcending the material plane. As a final goal one is expected to merge with the Absolute. In every human the true Self or Atman is living, which, though it is one with this Absolute, is now caught up in the relative reality of the space-time world. It is now searching for the way back to oneness. This would be no difficult task if we were not entangled by our improper deeds and passions, which cause us to fall back repeatedly into this world.

As long as we identify ourselves with this space-time world, which itself is only illusion or "*maya*" ruled by the cause and effect of our own deeds (karma), we remain bound by this illusion. Only someone who overcomes his ignorance and blindness to realize its unreality can free himself from his entanglement in this world of appearance. To do this and to free ourselves from the wheel of rebirth we normally have to go through the process of purification and knowledge leading to karma-free actions.

But there are also other means pointed out by various interpreters of the scriptures: above all the possibility of carrying out ritualistic religious activities. Every experienced traveler in India knows how much effort is put there into reducing karma either partly or wholly by such public ritualistic activities as: flower-offerings, renunciation vows, partial or complete oiling of stone figures, fire rituals, bathing or washing in holy rivers, sources or temples, pilgrimages to the residences of yogis, gurus, holy men or women, participation in regular holy festivals such as the *kumbamela* (an India-wide festival held every 12 years), proper treatment of dead bodies as well as dying at auspicious places (Benares or other holy places) or having one's ashes thrown into the Ganges etc.

Patanjali recommends in his sutras a kind of breathing technique that can reduce karmic ballast or at least protect one from new karma. Other holy persons recommend constant internal singing or reciting of mantras, as for instance the well-known mantras "*Hare Krishna, Hare Rama.*" The best means, however, practiced by many thousands, is considered to be remaining in the proximity of an ascetic monk living e.g. in a hole or cave and carrying out the life of a *sadhu*, i.e. someone without desires, living on whatever alms he receives.

The great saint *Ramakrishnan* recommended *karma-yoga* to his disciples. Here one may carry out normal business activities but practice complete devotion to God by meditating on His name and repeating it constantly, either silently or aloud. The closer one gets to God, the less karma can touch one. So any or all of these activities may lead finally to a state beyond karmic activities known as "*samadhi*" or merging with God. Because all karma dissolves finally in God [13].

An activity becoming more and more popular today is *bhakti-yoga*, which is seen as the most effective means of overcoming the wheel of eternal rebirth. Unconditional love of God as described in the Bhagavad-gita is the only way back to Him. And it is open to everyone, whether he is a Brahmin or someone without caste. Mutual love between God and His devotee leads to final unity by eliminating gradually the distance between them. But one may also be blessed by the higher mercy dispensed freely by a higher master or *avatar* and become immediately free of karma, have it reduced or the process speeded up.

However, the basic precondition even here, as emphasized again by *Patanjali*, remains the favorite old Indian postulate found also in Jainism and Buddhism, namely, fulfillment of the five vows: freedom from aggression, truthfulness, not stealing, non-attachment to possessions, sexual abstention.[14] *Patanjali* gives also an explanation of how the karmic seed stemming either from past lives ("earlier harvest") or from the present one ("present harvest") can be modified so as to eliminate its capacity to grow in a subsequent life. One can namely, through proper meditation practices, make the seed infertile and thus hinder not only a "bad harvest" but also any karmic "harvest" at all.[15]

13. Ramakrishna Math, p. 228 f.
14. Christopher Chapple in Hanson, p. 268
15. Doniger O'Flaherty, p. 246

Meditation seems in general to be the magic word of Indian wise men in approaching the divine sphere and facilitating final liberation ("*moksa*") from all earthly ballast, making it possible to devote oneself totally in one's present life to attaining unity with the eternal God.

The Indian saint Kabir

This great and wise Indian teacher lived in the 15th Century and was worshipped as a saint even during his own lifetime. Not only Hindus, Buddhists and Jains but even Moslems approached him for council on religious questions. He had already transcended the caste system, unifying in his teachings influences from the most diverse Indian sources. He reached the final postulate: "Karma comprises everything keeping us from finding God because it attaches us to something else."[16]

He saw three kinds of karma:

(1) *Sanchit*-karma is that good or bad karma that lies in the subconscious and is not manifested in our present life but will manifest itself in one of our coming lives. The spiritual master can take this karma upon himself if the devotee surrenders to him completely and puts himself under his protection. However, this is only possible under the condition that the disciple intends to take no new karma upon himself.

(2) *Prarabda*[??]-karma is manifested in one's present life on the basis of one's bad or good actions from previous lives. This karma also determines one's appearance, bodily stature, his health as well as the

16. Malhotra, p. 93

surroundings in which he is born and lives. All the things that will happen to him, whether good or bad, will take place without his being able to prevent them. These results from earlier causes can either lead to sorrow and suffering or to feelings of joy. The spiritual master will not be willing to eliminate this karma because the disciple would then not be able to attain the goal of his present life. But out of his groundless mercy the spiritual master may reduce his disciple's heavy burden.

The following incident is reported in this connection. A very scholarly man named Ramanand came to Kabir one day in great excitement, reporting that he had had the spontaneous remembrance of a previous life in which he had tied a man to his horse and dragged him to death. And suddenly he had become aware that that man had been reborn as well and had taken the position of the leading general of the army under the present king. He was now afraid that because of the unavoidable karmic law this general would cause his death by just such a fate, bringing about public shame for him. He asked the master to intervene in his favor, which the latter agreed to do. Kabir then visited this general, who had attained his high position on the basis of earlier good deeds, telling him of Ramanand's fears. The general responded that he also was well aware of this incident from his earlier life. Because of Kabirs intervention he agreed to not carry out the same type of retribution, but because of the karmic law he would be forced to kill Ramanand nevertheless. And in fact, during a later war campaign this general broke into Ramanand's house, killing him with a spear.

Another reported comment of Kabir's in a similar connection was that the afflicted person should be as happy as the debtor who had finally paid his debts.

(3) *Kriyaman*-karma is also known as free karma because it is karma that we have taken on in our present lives through voluntary acts of thinking, speaking and acting. Three-quarters of our actions and the events in our present life is determined by actions in previous lives while the remaining quarter is left to our own free disposition. Our way of carrying out this voluntary portion of our activities will again determine our reactions in later lives. The person who has understood what is going on here will manage his present life in such a way that he will not have to return with heavy karma but instead will open for himself the way back to his Creator.

For Kabir there is nothing that can dissolve our accumulated karma, at most there are ways, as we have seen, to reduce this karma. The only way to eliminate this karma completely is by experiencing the same suffering ourselves as we have dealt out to others. Nothing happens by chance because every thing is a result of things one has done in previous lives. It is also necessary for one to accept responsibility for one's own destiny by experiencing the consequences of one's acts. The law of karma is inevitable. The main guideline is that one should control one's thoughts, words and deeds in order not to gain new karma.

For such saints animals are just as much value as humans. For they have perhaps already been humans in earlier lives, perhaps even emperors, though they now have the bodies of chickens, cows. Or perhaps they have those of beasts of burden like mules or camels and are forced to slave beyond their actual strength. Now these souls have been reborn as animals because they acted wrongly at the time they themselves possessed a human body.[17]

Now we can see the reason for the Hindu's absolute vegetarianism: In this animal there may be the soul of a person, perhaps even of one who was very close to us before they died. Perhaps it is for a real Hindu – like for a Jain – an absolute sin to eat meat, since one may have to become an animal and likewise be eaten by a man or another animal in order to equalize the karma. Kabir refers us to the fact that one can load oneself with the least karma through vegetarian nutrition, in contrast to other diets.

We can see that the law of karma permeates the whole of everyday life in India. No one is willing to accept bad karma, since for carrying out bad deeds one will only have to reincarnate as some kind of animal or – even worse – one may have to transmigrate through the whole scale of different beings from the beginning, until one may some day again have the chance to become a human being - the only bodily form where one has the chance to get free of the wheel of rebirth.

Kabir also accepted the Vedic idea that the soul must live through 8,400,000 different types of living beings, among which also the plants are found, themselves alone making up 3 million types, while the insects, snakes and reptiles make up 2.7 million, birds and flying animals 1.4 million, water animals 0.9 million. The other animals including man,

17. Malhotra, p. 99

demigods and goddesses, demons, ghosts, fairies etc. then make up the remaining 0.4 million types.[18]

This concept puts very strong pressure on those planning evil actions because it could eventually cause them to accept karma – at worst even at the bottom of the evolutionary ladder, forcing them to start all over again and wait many more millions of lives before again receiving the almost unique gift of getting a human body. (Surely I am not the only one to notice that in India that hardly any adults are seen or heard laughing, except those who are not subject to or refuse to subject themselves to this karmic pressure. And this morphogenetic field also affects children.) It is therefore important to use the present life as a special opportunity to avoid accumulating karma again and thus take the path to final liberation. The wise man says quite unequivocally, "If one has all the riches of the world at his command and great knowledge to boot and does not know his own soul, he has lived in vain, for he has wasted his life."[19]

To sum up, we can say that Indian karmic thought is

18. Kirpal Singh, his son, Darshan Singh, and his son's successor, Rajinder Singh, follow in respect to rebirth, karma and support of karma dissolution for disciples in the footsteps of Kabir. They also think reincarnation of human souls in animal form to be possible. To demonstrate this point, Darshan Singh (p. 226) relates a story of Krishna (being a reincarnation of Vishnu). Krishna points with his finger at an insect crawling along the floor and says to Uddhava, "This creature was once Lord Indra, the god of thunder and rain. And often he has crawled in the dust like now. No living being can avoid this fate." That is, unless we live our lives in humility and love. Then we can overcome with the help of our spiritual master the eternal wheel of birth and rebirth and need never again fear being reborn, neither as a human nor as an animal.

19. Malhotra, p. 115

unthinkable without the concept of reincarnation. The main reference is to the causality of actions, which, if they intend something good, will bring about good reactions in a subsequent life and, if they are accompanied by evil thoughts and ego-centered feelings, will bring about unfavorable subsequent lives. Here there is an almost inevitable, though just, mechanism of retribution. Accumulated karma exists for the soul eternally as long as it fails to undertake the strenuous and exacting countermeasures necessary to free it from this entanglement. Still missing, however, is the rational explanation as to why this eternal wheel of rebirth for the souls – i.e. plants, animals and humans – exists at all, who has put it into movement and for what reason.

The revised karmic theory of Sri Aurobindo

"*Neo-Hinduism*", arising toward the end of the 19th and carrying over into the beginning of the 20th Century, was (according to Paul Hacker, who coined this name)[20] primarily influenced by three thinkers, namely Vivekananda, Radhakrishnan und Aurobindo. I would also like to add Krishnamurti and Yogananda to this list. They all have in common that they wrote their works primarily in English and traveled in the Western countries or at least were greatly influenced by thought from that area. As a result they naturally also spread this expanded Indian thought in Europe and America through their writings and/or lectures. They all concerned themselves with the new ideas of reincarnation and karma as propagated by Helena P. Blavatsky and Theosophy, clothing these ideas in more

20. Halbfass, p. 295

modern forms to help acquaint the Western reader with them.

Sri Aurobindo Ghosh says of Hinduism that this system was "only meant as an institution to turn the wheel of ignorance for all eternity, offering no other goal than finally the chance to jump off", and is "no philosophy with a real ontological basis."[21] He criticizes mainstream Hinduism for its "exaggerated individualism", because it has only been concerned with teaching the individual to free itself from the wheel of eternal rebirth. There is, according to him, in this system no gradual spiritual growth. Thus a "Mr. Smith" always remains a Mr. Smith, an eternal repetition of himself, even though his karmic characteristics may incarnate in new forms with different relationships and under different conditions.[22]

But in reality - and this is Sri Aurobindo's new approach - a new personality is born in each rebirth, i.e. no completely new Mr. Smith but rather a modified Mr. Smith, who does, of course, bring with him a great deal of his inherited past characteristics. However, he will have grown some spiritually. As we shall see later, this is just what Regression Therapy will tell us. Aurobindo also sees the fact that we usually do not remember previous lives as evidence that our soul improves from life to life. For memories from earlier lives would only "be in our way in developing other possibilities out of the depths of the mind." And referring to karma he explains, "The being of man, his nature and his living conditions are the result of his own inner and outer actions, not something accidental and inexplicable. He is that to

21. Hans-Peter Müller in Schmidt-Leukel, p. 64
22. Aurobindo I, p. 49

which he has made himself....Every person reaps what he sows. He profits from the good he does, he suffers from the bad."[23]

But Aurobindo turns against the cliche that a well-ordered previous life must reward us with an existence in pleasure and joy and a badly-lived life suffering and misfortune, while a life combining good and bad deeds brings forth a potpourri of both. For such a philosophy only leads us to live according to external criteria, not to grow internally, which latter is the real purpose of life. Such a philosophy – by transforming virtue into ego-centeredness – "replaces the proper motive for avoiding evil by a lower motive."[24]

Thus Sri Aurobindo has found the Achilles' heel of the whole Indian philosophical system. What good does it do to live a life free of karma by being outwardly sin-free and abiding rigorously by all regulations, while failing to grow within at all? Man must learn not to follow what is offered him from without as truth. Rather he should follow his own inner truth, which includes taking responsibility for his own actions, even if they conflict with other norms and even if he would have to accept negative consequences. "And what is true for my present life must be taken as true for the context of my actions and my self-realization throughout many lives."[25]

It is also self-contradictory to think that a scoundrel living in wealth and power could have earned this life by having carried out a previous life of purity and morality. To think this is possible is the sign of unhealthy judgment. For

23. quoted in Schmidt-Leukel, p. 66
24. quoted in Schmidt-Leukel, p. 68
25. quoted in Schmidt-Leukel, p. 69

"cosmic existence is no huge administration of universal justice with a cosmic law of reward and punishment as its mechanism."[26] Furthermore: If, however, the fundamental truth of our existence is spiritual and not mechanical, then it must be our Self, our soul which fundamentally determines its own evolution. It is not imaginable that our spirit is a machine in the hands of karma, a slave of previous actions in this life.[27] For him karma is a valid law, but one connected with the spiritual purpose of self-realization and subject to the Creator's higher will and intention. And he mentions also already the word "love" as a medium for the soul's development, though this is not a central point of his philosophical considerations.

What is especially positive about his approach is, however, the fact - and here he anticipates Regression Therapy - that he transfers to the soul of man the freedom to decide its own fate. Karma is thus no longer something good or evil attached from without. Rather the soul itself accepts its own responsibility, using karma only as a stepping-stone to perfection. The empirical results of Regression Therapy support his courageous thoughts and will surely awaken many readers and encourage them to study more deeply his integral philosophy.

He also thinks that these insights cannot be gained through rational knowledge alone, but require spiritual experience. Therapeutic reincarnation sessions in the alpha-state make such spiritual experiences possible, as we shall see later.

A further strong criticism of the Hindu system of karma

---

26. quoted in Schmidt-Leukel, p. 71
27. Aurobindo I, p. 49

is that it is morally grim because it knows nothing of the Christian and Buddhist ideal of empathy and mercy. The law of karma is as a merciless *lex talionis* (law of retribution) a godless codex of primitive and barbaric justice.[28]

It is understandable that Hinduism would not take such blows lying down, for which reason Aurobindo's criticism has found in Indian thought little resonance to date. But still another thinker was to come whose voice would be heard more clearly: Sai Baba.

Sai Baba and Karma

Although there are many interesting statements by other Indian spiritual masters on karma, I would like to close this short introduction to the concept of karma in India with a few relevant thoughts of Sai Baba. The main purpose of this introduction is not to give an encyclopedic survey of the subject, but only to present the reader with some different perspectives on karma and to stimulate him to his own thoughts respecting the findings of Regression Therapy.

Sai Baba, whom I have personally had the pleasure of meeting, says of himself, "I am God." However he immediately adds, "You, too, are God. You just don't know it." He also says that there is no karma binding him to this world, just his love. I may state already at this point that, after Christ, it is Sai Baba who most consequently emphasizes the role of love – and not only love of God – for our inner evolution. Karma means for him human activity, and one can do nothing, nothing at all, which is without consequences.

---

28. quoted in Hummel, p. 53

The law of karma he formulates in a way already familiar to us at this point: If you do good, the results will be positive, if you do bad, the consequences will be bad for you.[29] This is, as he says, the whole truth of the matter, which one should never try to ignore. For many centuries this law has, he says, been ignored by the Occident, or at least it refused to take karmic reactions into consideration, although Jesus Christ also taught this law. And the consequences of this lack have been catastrophic.

Everyone is the master of his own destiny through his actions. Whatever one has done in the past, it has also its effects in the present. And everything that we do in the present will determine our future lives. But it is God who decides where, when and in which way the consequences of our actions come into play. However, God will act in such a way that the free will of man is not restricted. At the same time man will learn through the consequences of his actions – this is the meaning of the word [to gain] "experience". Here the human being is considered to have full freedom in his actions.

The situations in which the consequences come into play are seen to be determined by a Higher Power, which Sai Baba calls "God." The distribution of the karmic law is dependent on His final decision, although He does take into consideration the free will of man, who has put himself in this situation by his own thought, speech and actions.

Here man is no longer the passive instrument of the

---

29. v. Stepski-Doliwa I, p. 80. In the following exposition I draw, unless explicitly stated otherwise, on the elaborations of Sai Baba compiled by Stephan von Stepski-Doliwa (p. 79-84).

mechanically turning wheel of eternal rebirth but is simply being supported by God in the development of his soul. God is responsible for preparing the learning steps for the soul of man in accordance with his karma. If we consider the fact, as Sai Baba says, that we ourselves are God – without, however, normally being aware of this fact – it could be that we by attaining a higher knowledge are also able ourselves to determine at least in part the conditions for karmic retribution in our next life.

These are courageous thoughts leading far beyond present Hindu thinking. And they are also thoughts that have been confirmed in Regression Therapy, as we will later see. Sai Baba, who is worshipped by millions as a living God, sees a higher purpose in the karmic process. Karma is the inner breath of life, he says. Without the law of cause and effect the world would be meaningless and God something like a drunken player. God is however perfect justice, the real purpose of your existence. Because of this righteousness and justice karma may exist. And in order to fulfill your karmic purpose you have been born and you will be reborn. Therefore your life, every life has a meaning. Therefore you have attained salvation from the very beginning.[30]

God loves man, and no man can therefore be lost – in the long run. Everyone determines under his own direction how quickly he may be united with God, i.e. how fast he is able to dissolve his karmic entanglement and gain no more negative karma. Sai Baba has coined a new concept of karma, namely *niskaama-karma*, referring to a stage when we are no longer concentrating on the fruits of our actions. Then we are already in a state of inner union with God and

30. v. Stepski-Doliwa II, p. 45

act in the proper manner through His support and for His purposes. Therefore we are one with His will.

And in order to become aware of our actual unity with God there are three necessary steps: First, one must become aware that one's activities are subject to the law of karma. The second step consists in only acting positively in order to attain a good result. The third step consists of no longer thinking of the results of one's deeds but simply offering everything to God. On this last stage one no longer acts out of one's own will and for one's own purposes. Thus the law of karma is in effect only until "free will" is transformed into "God's will."

Love as the key to liberation from the wheel of eternal rebirth

We have seen that the concept of love as the actual motor of karma is gaining more and more acceptance even in India. What caused the thought of karma to arise in the first place was the question why some have to suffer while others are allowed to enjoy their lives in relative harmony. Why is one person confronted with bad luck and illness while someone else may be healthy and free of misfortunes? Originally, because there seemed to be no clear answer to this question, the "gods" were blamed for fortune and misfortune. Someone who was unfortunate could suppose himself to have angered the gods or caused their displeasure by not paying sufficient respect or not carrying out enough offering ceremonies. Therefore great emphasis was laid on carrying out offerings and paying respect. This attitude is still found clearly in the Vedas as well as in most original religions.

But there is also another variation: Not the gods

determine good and evil, but ghosts and/or demons that have a positive or negative disposition toward one and can thus cause joy or suffering. Therefore it is necessary to bring them offerings or to obey their commands. Such invisible powers reveal themselves through numerous omens: birds behaving in a certain way or the words of mediums etc. The attempt was thus made to make invisible influences responsible for one's destiny. The ominous meting out of destiny became however gradually more anthropogenic, until suddenly the *Upanishads* developed the idea that a person can himself be the cause of his own destiny without having to refer to an invisible power. This was the birth-hour of karma.

Many original religions contained the concept of gods, demigods, demons and ghosts. The concept of a single God (*Echnaton*) arose first temporarily in Egypt, then permanently with the Jews (*Abraham*). Meanwhile in India man's destiny was becoming more and more his own individual responsibility. The concept of karma arose. But if the idea of karma is only applied to one life, then many questions are left open. So the idea of reincarnation offered the logical answer: Whatever appears to have no karmic cause in one's present life can be attributed to an earlier life. Not God or ghosts etc. were now seen as the causes, but the person himself through his actions in the same or in earlier lives.

About 450 B.C. we see this concept spreading out increasingly, and from 200 B.C. on it became more and more predominant in Indian thought, resulting in a true explosion in karmic philosophy. And from about 0 B.C. on innumerable philosophical systems were constructed and old texts were revised in light of these new ideas, being then "backdated" and attributed to the religious founders. Besides quite a few absurd constructions, there were also numerous philosophical ideas of great depth that found their expression in holy texts, and these were subsequently improved and repeatedly revised and deepened.

All of India, whether Hindus, Jains or Buddhists, had now come under the spell of the concept of karma. So everyone knew that all joy and suffering was self-induced – a result of one's previous actions. A miserly, hard-hearted person might have been rich because he had done something good in an earlier life. Even so, he could calculate - if his ego allowed – that he would be punished for his present misdeeds in his next life by being reborn as a beggar or worse, perhaps even as a dog. But if he then acted according to moral principles and the proper scriptures, in his subsequent life he could again attain a position of wealth etc.

This concept of karma is thus still lacking the idea of a gradual upward progression from life to life. One seemed to be bound to an eternally rotating wheel. And karma was the right "fuel for samsara".[31] Every wish and every desire expressed in word or deed would necessarily have its consequences, if not in this life, then in a coming life. Thus it seemed almost impossible for someone to escape this cycle of eternal rebirths, unless one fulfilled the many required rules and regulations. The main or only way out would be to renounce all personal desires, whether positive or negative.

And renunciation has since then – even up to today – appeared for most Indians the only escape. If one lusts for

31. Hummel, p. 45

anything whatsoever, one will be condemned to renewed incarnation. If one happens to be a virtuous and God-loving person who would never do evil to anyone, one can attain a pleasant coming life but still never escape the wheel of rebirth. And someone with passionate desires and inconsiderate behavior throughout his life could calculate the sufferings awaiting him in his coming life!

Indian thought had consolidated itself within the masses as an inescapable, almost insoluble chaining mechanism, chaining one to the cycle of eternal rebirth. This burden of karma caused a depressive fatalism to spread out among the population. Every kind of ill fate was self-induced by ignorance or stupidity in an earlier life. Repeatedly great and wise teachers have spoken out against this fatalism, offering instruction to facilitate liberation from samsara but without making much effect on the overriding fatalistic mentality.[32] Even today the Indian population is still stuck in a kind of "karmic depression." Someone can fall dead on Indian streets and no one will take notice or take care of the body, as I myself once experienced in Puna: A bicycle-driver fell over dead in the street and the traffic continued on peacefully around the dead body. Just as little concern is shown for someone lying in pain at the side of the street obviously in need of medical attention.

This mistaken conception of karma has caused a widespread feeling of indifference toward the suffering of others: "What problem is it of mine that this person is suffering. He has brought this upon himself in an earlier life, so it is his own business and none of mine. I have my

32. Radhakrishnan said that Hinduism had become a message of despair and fatalism instead of a message of hope (Hummel, p. 51).

own destiny to take care of, and no one will take care of me when I lie suffering some day at the side of the street." This karmic attitude shows a lack of empathy, and every lack of empathy is also a sign of lack of love. Mother Theresa wanted to show Indians through her loving care and her loving actions that love of mankind is the important thing –important also in leading one to God.

The law of karma, when understood as in the present way in India, leads to apathy, fatalism, hard-heartedness and indifference toward others and their destiny. But this great lesson, namely that karma actually leads us to love – i.e. that it is not in opposition to, but actually stands for and helps us finally to attain love itself – this lesson is still very far beyond most Indians' horizon. For everyone who is indifferent toward the destiny of other also commits an offense against love itself, causing him to gain more negative karma.[33]

In this way one is always in a kind of karma-trap. The dullness stemming from lack of empathy and love causes new karma. The Indians are today, in contrast e.g. to the period of the *Kama-sutra*, exceedingly prudish. For all regulations that are supposed to lead to liberation from the wheel of eternal rebirth include sexual renunciation.[34]

---

33. Gina Cerminara, who compiled Edgar Cayce's thoughts on karma, says that indifference toward the suffering of others is in itself a sin worthy of karmic reactions (p. 257).
34. Even tantric sexual practices are actually aimed at raising kundalini and thus experiencing higher levels of consciousness and closeness to God. In the West people like to practice this in seminars meant also to increase sexual enjoyment. But in India itself such practices, although they are also taught sometimes, are rare, being generally considered more a form of temptation and renewed entanglement in karma.

Sexual lust is a guarantee for a renewed earthly life under unfavorable conditions. Sexual enjoyment, which in other areas - for instance Africa – is seen as helping in many ways to support the joy of life, is considered improper in India.

Sexuality – a gift of creation to humanity, not only in order to produce children, but also to be enjoyed for its own sake – is an expression of pure joy of life. In India this is made impossible by the predominant, depressive philosophy of karma. For in reality a loving person does not gain karma, no matter how much he is attached to sexuality. Rather he will gain more karma through the decision – even if it is on karmic philosophical grounds – to withhold love from his loving partner.

In India there must be a great change of mind in respect to karma in order to produce joy of life among the people. Sexual self-restriction cannot open the gates to liberation from rebirth, but rather practical, unrestricted love of one's neighbor. As we have seen, Aurobindo recognized the desperate situation caused by the Indian understanding of karma and offered a new understanding, which was however only known to the philosophically interested persons, not to the masses.

Many other Indian thinkers, swamis and gurus have also found concepts to liberate the people from such depression, connected them to a gradual improvement of the soul from life to life through good behavior and proposed very different means of doing so. But it seems to me that Sai Baba was the first to give people the real key to release themselves from the wheel of eternal rebirth. This key is called LOVE. This means not only love of God, as postulated in the *Bhagavad-gita*, but love of all living beings, humans, animals, plants, God – simple, unrestricted love.

This key to escaping from eternal rebirth can be attained by everyone.

It is true that the karmic law returns to every person what he has caused himself. If one has caused a great amount of love to take place in life, one will also receive love in his next life again. At some time he will attain complete love in his thinking, speaking and acting and will not need to return to the earth again to perfect himself still further in this love. He will be complete. The whole meaning of life on earth, including the law of karma, is only to become pure love.

Thus karma is no longer an end in itself, but only a means to becoming pure love. This is, as far as I can see, Sai Baba's great contribution, and his liberating message is spreading itself further and further. It can become a wonderful message also for Indians, perhaps just as effective as that of the other great preacher of love, Jesus, who gave us the great commandment, "Love thy neighbor as thyself." He meant by this nothing other than what Sai Baba says: "Become completely love, be love in all you think, you speak and do."

No longer does karma chain one eternally to the eternal wheel of rebirth, but offers instead liberation through love. Karma is no longer the enemy of mankind but its best friend. This karma is no longer a "brake" for reunification with God but, as we will see later, its "accelerator."

And Regression Therapy leads us to exactly the same results. As we will see in "Part 3" of the present book, the subconscious revelations of clients guided back through previous lives prove karmic entanglements to arise only from hard-heartedness, i.e. from not having accepted the law of love. And the law of karma is the instrument that teaches us to love. Not until we experience in a subsequent life the hard-heartedness that we have caused by our actions do we gradually recognize the value of love. Karma is therefore the most wonderful instrument toward "becoming love."

Part Two

A Brief Introduction to Practical Regression Therapy

Look for a therapist who will join you in searching for your truth and will therefore find it because he has already found his and is living it.

(*Sai Baba*)

Before turning to the karmic causes for different symptoms, it is important to explain briefly the method of Regression Therapy used here. This type of therapy takes advantage of the fact that our subconscious stores everything ever experienced by us, whether in this life, in the womb of our mother or in earlier existences. There is so-called "cognitive storing" of information and storing in the *emotional body*, both of which accompany the soul on all its travels through different lives in different bodies.

In order to access this information we have to put the client into the so-called "*alpha-state*", a stage of consciousness attained between the waking, or "beta-state," and the sleeping state. In the alpha-state the analytical, controlling left hemisphere is turned off and the right hemisphere of the brain containing the subconscious is turned on as much as possible.

The Tibetans used hyperventilation and the Indians generally yoga and meditation techniques to do the same. We in America and Europe prefer the hypnosis technique or the countdown relaxation technique.

Even before accepting an appointment, on the phone or in a pre-talk we attempt to establish whether such a treatment is possible for the client – whether immediately or at a later time. The only restrictions are for those already under psychiatric care or treatment, in which case the permission of the current therapist or medical doctor is required to avoid disturbing a treatment already in progress.

At the first appointment a complete *anamnesis* is carried out, so the therapist can get a very clear picture not only of the symptoms of the particular problem to be treated, but also of the total life situation, e.g. life history, family, occupation, general status of present or past illnesses of the client. Then we explain to the client how the therapy will be carried out. If the decision has been made by both client and therapist to begin immediately with the therapy, the client is asked to lie or sit in a comfortable position.

As soon as the client has been put in the alpha-state he is led in his imagination over a meadow to a healing source, where he is asked to feel the healing power of the water while drinking. And later, after his return from his earlier lives, he will take a healing bath in this source. Finally, we have him imagine a bed of clouds, in which he is asked to lie down and to feel himself clothed and protected by divine energy. At this point he meets his – generally "invisible" – *Higher Self*, perhaps experienced as an "angel" or a "guide." The Higher Self knows everything about the client, even about his earlier lives, for it represents his own higher knowledge, the direct contact between him and the divine sphere. As a part of the divine sphere it is also all-knowing.

The client asks now the Higher Self to lead him to the source of the problem or symptom. The Higher Self takes his hand, leading him to one of many gates in a long wall of clouds, behind which he finds his present or one of his past lives. Here the theme of the present sitting or "session" is precisely formulated, and it is also determined that the client upon a count of three will find himself in the life in question. It will be exactly one day previous to the beginning of an event important for the development of his present symptom or problem. In most cases we will find that we are in a *life as a victim*. The client discovers then who and where he is, what his name is, what country he is in, if he is married or single, what his profession is etc.

Then he is led to the event of the following day. Here he experiences the cause for his present problem or symptom. For example, if he suffers in his present life from asthma – just as in the first case following in "Part 3" – he may experience himself as a "witch" at the stake and feel himself being smothered by smoke, even before the flames can destroy his body. This re-experiencing is not the same as in reality but as in a mental form, i.e. tears may run, but seldom is pain actually felt. Perhaps, depending on the decision of the therapist, a visit to the period in the beyond - i.e. the period between lives – will also be on the agenda, because the events that are experienced there – as we will see later - may be very revealing.

Brought again before the wall of clouds, the client learns from the Higher Self that some participants in his just re-experienced life have also re-appeared in his present life. (Souls from the different bodies throughout many lives meet again and again, until they have found harmony among themselves.) Afterwards the Higher Self is asked if there still are one or more earlier lives in which other causes for the present symptoms may be found. If the answer is yes, the process begins once more, and the search begins again for a "life as a victim", another life of suffering and retribution.

If all the necessary causes have been found in lives as a victim and re-experienced – usually in an emotional way – then the Higher Self will be asked before the gate of clouds to now take the client to the life or lives where the actual cause of suffering can be found. The Higher Self then leads the client in a previous so-called "life as a perpetrator", in which he has caused other persons suffering or pain. Here the actual or primary cause is found for the symptom or problem later manifesting itself in lives as a victim and still felt as a symptom or problem in his present one - a life as a victim or a life in its aftermath.

In such a *life as a perpetrator*, the soul has carried out an action making it not only guilty for others but also in its own eyes. This feeling of guilt often remains present in the subconscious over many lives and can develop into a guilt complex of unknown origin, leading to depression, inferiority complexes and helper syndromes. Therefore it is very important also to experience the life as a perpetrator to free the person permanently from his guilty feelings during the dissolution process. This will also help him to forgive more easily those who have caused him pain and suffering during his lives as a victim. Now he may understand that there is a higher meaning and a just purpose and that nothing happens in accordance with the law of karma that the person has not caused himself.

After re-experiencing all the relevant earlier lives chosen by the Higher Self, the client is led to the so-called *Mountain of Revelation*. From this higher vantage point the earlier lives spread out before him can be compared with his present life. Recognizing their interconnection through the law of karma - which he now accepts as being just – helps him to see their connections to his present life.

After that, the Higher Self gives him a *Golden Cup* like a golden chalice with a liquid containing the power of love, forgiveness and dissolution of suffering and guilt. The client takes this cup into his life as a perpetrator and asks all those who have suffered because of him for forgiveness. Then he offers the perpetrator – who he was himself – the cup, thus releasing himself from all guilt. After that he takes the cup into each of the lives as a victim discovered in the session, forgiving all of those who have brought him suffering and pain, finally offering the cup to the person he himself was then, thus freeing his earlier self from all suffering and pain. He then takes the cup into his present life, where he offers it to everyone he now knows to have been either a victim or perpetrator in one of his earlier lives, forgiving them or asking them for forgiveness for his former or present offenses against them. Finally he stands in front of himself and forgives himself for all the evils done to others in earlier lives or in the present one.

As the next step the Higher Self gives him a large open *pinecone* into whose spaces he now stuffs everything he would like to give up, including his feelings of guilt. The filled cone is then burned with all its contents in a bright fire and all stuffed-in items are returned to the original source of all love. Then the client formulates his resolution affirmation, beginning as follows: "I am free of ...." after this affirmation is repeated several times, he is led back to the bed of clouds and finally back to the healing source and from there back into the here and now.

The client generally possesses a double consciousness while standing in front of the cloud gate or before the Higher Self or on the Mountain of Revelation. He realizes that he is presently in the office of his therapist – and at the same time he is experiencing all those earlier lives. But in addition to this on the Mountain of Revelation a third – and higher – consciousness is added.

Thus many clients experience Regression Therapy as a

kind of "*initiation*" into a new and extended understanding of themselves and of existence as a whole. Afterwards one lives in a more conscious and fulfilling way - somewhat like those who, having experienced clinical death, often return as "reborn" persons. For this reason regression therapists think that it is unfortunate that only their clients and patients get this experience instead of its being open for all interested parties.

Such a Regression Therapy session may last from three to six hours. There is, however, the advantage that generally no further appointment is necessary: either the problem has been solved or the symptom has found a spontaneous dissolution or the begin of a gradual one.

Exact data are generally a matter for the left hemisphere of the brain - which we try to minimize in Regression Therapy. In spite of this names and dates often turn up in an imprecise or incomplete form. Occasionally, however, they are surprisingly exact and even accompanied by the date of birth, making them checkable in old registries. Also, many souls may not have been aware of the exact year in their earlier life, or of the name of the ruling king or the country (the present names or countries may not have even existed at that time). In general one can say: the deeper the alpha-state, the more correct the data. Inexactness in factual data has, however, no influence on the effectiveness of Regression Therapy. And "Cleopatras", "Napoleons" or "Shakespeares" never turn up in Regression Therapy – these are generally the product of worthless pseudo-recollections or of the suggestive hints of would-be psychics to stimulate the narcissistic egos of their clients.

Most people expect therapy to be a long-term process of somatic, psychosomatic or psychic correction of an ailing or dysfunctional condition. In Regression Therapy it may, however, only take a single session of a few hours to attain partial or complete correction.

The cases described in the following "Part 3" can only offer a small sampling among hundreds of similar cases treated in my practice with Regression Therapy. The present names of the clients have, of course, been changed to maintain anonymity, though earlier names have not. The sessions are repeated "as is" (i.e. as recorded by hand or, whenever possible, by tape).

Part Three

The karmic causes of symptoms as brought to light by Regression Therapy

KARMIC AND PSYCHOSOMATIC SYMPTOMS

1. Why she chose to be burned at the stake as a witch (Asthma)

Angelica is a woman of forty-four years of age in her second marriage. Her present husband is a doctor. From childhood on she has often had to gasp for air. Attacks of incessant coughing were also one of her symptoms. Medicine for asthma and pollen-allergy was prescribed for her from the age of 15. When hay was thrown on her at the age of 16, she experienced a state of panic. Asthma and attacks of suffocation occurred almost constantly, and the pollen season was a nightmare. Later she also became allergic to dust and feathers. At 36 she caught tuberculosis of the lungs. Although her asthmatic attacks worsened, she could not give up smoking, so she usually – as she herself expressed it – held a cigarette in one hand while keeping her asthma spray ready in the other. Furthermore she suffered from arachno-phobia (spider phobia), fear of heights and a strong dislike of crowds.

As she was in training as a regression therapist, I decided to use her case in a demonstration for the other trainees. After I had put her in the alpha-state and the Higher Self had led her to the Gate of Clouds, we went through a life to find the cause for her present asthma. Upon going through the gate she found herself in Normandy (France) in the year 1346, claiming to be Susanne Brisson, 23 years of age, who sold herbs to make a living for herself and her children. At this moment there were numerous militiamen with her in the mill she was presently visiting. Accusing her of having poisoned the cows of the area, they arrested her and took her to the city.

Being asked by me about the reasons for these accusations, she answered as follows: She had been having an affair for the past two years with an aristocrat of the city, Jean-Jacques Bernadotte, son of the Lord of Rennes, who she had met in the forest and who had visited her often in her out-of-the-way house at the edge of the forest. But secretly she was in love with another man from whom she had already had two children, but who had abandoned her. She had not been able to love Jean-Jacques and had therefore stopped letting him into her house. He seemed to be taking revenge on her for that now.

The city militia, clothed in coats of mail and armed with spears, took her to prison. She was very fearful because her girlfriend had already been accused of witchcraft and publicly burned at the stake. The next day, a man dressed in black read the accusation, in which she was accused of having an evil eye and bewitching men. She was also supposed to have recently cast her eye on a woman, causing her to have a miscarriage. She was claimed to have bewitched by magic the cows of the area, too, afflicting them with an illness from which many had died. Thus "proven" a witch, she was to be burned at the stake. Then she was pulled by the hair downstairs to her cell, still loudly proclaiming her innocence.

Angelica related all of these incidents as if she were experiencing them at the moment. Her face was locked in a grimace of terror and shock while tears flowed down her cheeks.

Then she described the day of her execution. She was acquainted with one of the guards who pulled her out of her cell and commanded her to put on a white gown. He nodded to her request to take care of her two little children.

She was then led onto the market place. There the crowd began to cheer. Screaming insults, they seemed to all be enjoying the spectacle. Priests on the steps of the church, and she was shocked to see Jean-Jacques among them, her last hope for freedom because of his influence.

While she was being led to the stake, a sympathizing priest whispered to her that she would soon be free, since the fire would drive the devil out of her. She was then taken to a platform where she was bound to the stake. Another priest demanded loudly that she confess her sins. But Susanne just spit in reply at him, which was answered by the jeering screams of the mob. At that point the drums began to roll. She glanced at Jean-Jacques, who was staring at the ground. Then she could already feel the flames crawling up her body.

At this point Angelica began to cough. In my therapeutic sessions I have seen a great number of asthmatics that have had to experience death at the stake. The flames enveloping the body from below consume so much oxygen that the person usually suffocates before the flames can destroy the body.

Suddenly Suzanne found herself outside the body, viewing the whole scene from above. She looked into the still horrified faces of the spectators. Thereafter she was flying to her house at the edge of the forest, where she saw the miller's wife taking care of her children. Then she was surrounded by light-bodies, among whom she recognized both her parents. She was then "led into the light", as she described it, and came into a great hall. There she recognized other figures, i.e. souls, who altogether formed a great family, of which she was also a member. A wise old man named Abraham took her in his arms. A woman took her by the hand. To her question about the reason for the cruel experience the woman replied that she herself had already chosen the fate of being burned at the stake before her birth as Suzanne, as she had in an earlier life also burned people or had had them burned.

From this birth as Suzanne, Angelica was again lead to the Gate of Clouds, where the Higher Self revealed to her that both her children from that life were again her children in this life, that Jean-Jacques was her second husband and the priest that she had spat at was her first husband. Later she reported that whenever she saw either of these husbands, she always felt a tightening of the chest and had to cough or clear her throat. *So other persons having to do with the causes for symptoms from an earlier life can also trigger the same response in one's present life.*

But now I requested her to ask the Higher Self to lead her into the life where she had caused the burning of others. She sees herself now as a Germanic warrior named Igurk in the year 572. He admittedly has taken many women by force, killed many persons and otherwise often plundered and razed different places. At the moment he and others are again preparing to plunder a village – out of boredom. He describes how he, along with 12 or 13 other warriors, attack the village. The people scatter in panic, while the attackers plunder, destroy and raze the houses. He sets the torch himself to a hut and hears suddenly the cry of a child. This cry haunts him from then on, causing him to end his life as a warrior out of regret for his deeds and finally to become a beggar.

After death he stands beside his earthly body, afraid of confronting those who he had pained or even killed in that life. And when I ask him, "What would you say if you looked back and said, 'I will never again....'?", he answers "I will never again cause pain to others. I will always show respect towards the life of others and help the weak and needy."

On the Mountain of Revelation Angelica learns that the cause of her asthma has now been revealed and that it is therefore not necessary to visit another life in this connection, but that the cause for her hay fever could be investigated in another life. Her fear of crowds also stems from this life as Suzanne. With the Golden Cup in hand, Angelica now goes into this life as Igurk, begs forgiveness from all those to whom Igurk has caused suffering. And gives the cup also to Igurk himself and absolves him of his guilt. Finally Angelica takes the cup into her life as Suzanne, forgives all her enemies as well as the members of the jeering crowd, gives it also to Suzanne herself and releases her from all her suffering experiences in that life.

Then she takes into her present life the cup of love, forgiveness and release from suffering and guilt, giving it to her two husbands, who she forgives for their earlier acts against her, and to her children, who she asks for forgiveness for their suffering, and finally to herself, who she forgives for all the suffering caused others as Igurk. She also releases her suffering from the life as Suzanne.

She then puts everything of which she would like to free herself at this moment into the pine-cone, saying, "I free myself of all my lung problems, my constant need to clear my throat, my fear of men and of greater crowds. I free myself of the need to punish others and myself. I free myself from all my guilt feelings."

After returning to the present moment, she suddenly cries, "I can breathe again freely!" It was the first time for weeks that her respiratory system was free again. She felt as if a great weight had been taken from her chest. Two weeks later I called her at home to ask her again about her asthma. She told me that two days after that session, her respiratory system had worsened again somewhat but that it had since then been improving again day by day so that she was again completely free of asthma. Nevertheless she wanted to have another session at the next opportunity in order to free herself from her hay fever. But this was not so pressing, it being winter at the time.

The woman who had taken Suzanne by the hand in the beyond said to her that she had chosen her death at the stake herself. When we are in "the beyond", in the intermediate period between two earthly lives, and have sinned greatly against love, we feel the need to make up for our misdeeds. We learn from our instructors there that we can integrate such loveless misbehavior into our scope of experience by living through a similar loveless event which we have caused to a victim.

So we can only grow and clear our karmic account if all wrongs that we commit are also committed against us. After gaining this insight we can finally realize the need to allow the karmic clearing process to happen to us. We are then offered the decision whether to have this experience in the immediately following life or in a later one (because other learning steps may be more pressing at the moment).

Now in this regression therapy we concentrated on asthma. Her hay fever symptoms had to wait for another regression.

2. Why she wanted to be raped as a woman (Hay fever).

It was however to be a whole year until Angelica would

discover the reasons for her hay fever. This took place in a supervisory seminar in which the aspirants for a diploma as regression therapists were to prove their abilities and learn new techniques. She said that since the first Regression Therapy session she had had for the first time the feeling that she had two lungs and her asthma had not turned up again She had in the meantime passed her healing practitioner (non-medical practitioner) examination.

The relationship to her husband had already been worsening for many years, so she still resisted his touching her, even though she had forgiven him for having been in that former life her lover, then betrayer. Though in such cases relationships are often re-harmonized, she had even decided to separate from her husband, expecting to soon be able to stand on her own two feet as a healing practitioner and regression therapist.

She had also realized that her distaste for the sound of drums stemmed from hearing them while being burned at the stake. *Sensory experiences connected with such horrifying experiences often remain in later lives inexplicable stimulants for aversion or discomfort.* Her pollen allergy began at the beginning of March with birch, worsened in May-July with grasses and continued in a milder form on through August and September. These attacks had begun with an attack of panic in a haystack at the age of 15, the year she met her first husband, and had worsened after she married him at the age of 16.

Four diploma aspirants under my supervision and occasional intervention carried out the following Regression Therapy session, while the other aspirants listened carefully and took notes. Some parts will be quoted word-for-word.

Angelica's Higher Self was asked to lead her to the causal

life for her present hay fever, and she suddenly found herself as Marianca about 1800 in Poland. Her parents had a farm and six children, of whom Marianca was the oldest. She was waiting for a rendezvous with her boyfriend in the haystack behind the house, when three young seasonal workers discovered her. They pressed her against the haystack, two of them taking off her clothes and holding her while the third abused her. Frozen with fear, Marianca was afraid to call for help, fearing they might kill her. After one of the three had raped her, they left laughing. She felt as if she had died and blamed herself for the incident, because she should not have been there. Dressing again, she ran home in shame.

She vowed never again to have anything to do with men, not even with her boyfriend, and not to tell her parents anything about the event. Whenever she saw the young men afterwards, they would laugh at her, making her feel ashamed but also filling her with excessive hate. Luckily she was not pregnant, but her self-esteem had been totally destroyed. Withdrawing into herself, she broke contact with the outside world, became despondent and was thought to be crazy. Longing to die, she left home for a life of begging, wandering by day and sleeping wherever she could at night. Finally, hungry and exhausted, she lay down and died.

"I will count now to three, and then you will have just died. 1 - 2 - 3.... You have just died. What do you see?"

"I am sitting."

"Can you feel your body?"

"Yes, I can feel myself again. My body is lying there very still. Now I am really free."

"What do you see?"

"Two beings are coming."

"Do you know these beings?"

"No."

"What do they look like? Describe them, please."

"They look like normal persons. They are happy. I feel very happy, too. I feel so light. I am simply happy....I am shining so brightly....Everything is shining here so brightly, and I am full of light. I have a body completely full of light."

Are you going anywhere?

Yes, home.

Where is your home?

It's just like being at home. Many people are here. They are laughing a lot.

Are they glad that you have come?

Yes, that's true too. But they are simply happy. They are like that. They are all very happy.

Is there anyone you know?

They all seem familiar.

What are you doing there?

I am now at home. I am now relaxing.

What does it look like where you are now?

Everything is easier and more fun here. I hear laughter everywhere. The people are happy.

How are the people dressed?

They have flowing robes on. They are white, everything is full of light.

What does the world there look like? Are there flowers?

There is everything here that there is on earth.

Animals, too?

I don't see any.

What are you occupying yourself with?

I still feel the anger in my stomach about everything that

happened. About those three men.

Why do you feel this anger now?

Because I am free. It is not pain, just anger.

Can you talk with someone about it?

Yes, I can talk about it, and they listen.

What do they say?

They say I shouldn't have killed the life in me.

What could you have done better?

I should have felt. I should have felt the pain.

Was it important for you to feel this pain?

Because I didn't feel it, I died inside. One should feel one's feelings.

Was it something like a test that you experienced on earth?

Yes.

And did you pass this test?

No.

Do you have to repeat the test, or what do they tell you?

I don't need to repeat it, but I have to look at everything very carefully from the vantage point here.

Do you have a teacher who speaks to you there?

Yes, there are three teachers.

Do you know one of them? Have you met one of them before?

I don't know. But they all seem very familiar.

How can you look at the former events?

I experience them again. I experience the emotions now that I didn't feel then. I feel the guilt, and then I feel the love.

The feelings of guilt that you felt there, were they justified?

No, feelings of guilt are never justified. Love heals everything.

Do you still have that feeling of anger now?

No.

If you said, "I will never again....", what would you say now?

I will never again be pushed into a corner, never again die within. I will never again keep everything shut up within me.

Now Angelica is led back in front of the Gate of Clouds to her Higher Self:

Ask your Higher Self why you had to experience this fate.

I was supposed to learn even in deep pain still to remain aware.

Is there anyone from that earlier life again in your present life?

Only my son....

Ask your Higher Self whether there are still other earlier lives containing a reason why you have to suffer from hay fever today.

No.

Ask your Higher Self why you had to die of hunger there.

I died of hunger because I didn't want to eat any more.

Why did you have to experience all that as Marianca?

I had to feel how it is to be so helpless. I was supposed to learn that one should not misuse power [in the life as a perpetrator].

And then Angelica was led to the life that was the cause for her having to suffer the life as Marianca:

She sees herself as the thirty-two year-old merchant and ship-owner Igor in the year 1234. Besides all kinds of wares he also is carrying three 14 to 15 year-old girls, who he hopes to sell somewhere. Their parents sold them to him. Igor enjoys watching as the twelve men on board rape these girls. He feeds on their fear. The girls have to clean the ship during the day. He himself has also a 16 year-old girl named

Plischka, who he also has bought. She is pretty, but he doesn't love her. She rejects him, too, but she dares not showing her feelings, as he kills anyone who doesn't like him or leaves them somewhere on land, as soon as he is tired of them.

Led to the end of his life, he sees himself still on his ship – now as a bad-tempered old man with a pain in his left leg. Two men have to apply cold poultices to his leg. Asked how he found his life as a whole, he answers, "Great." But now – sensing himself to be close to death - he has the uncomfortable feeling that perhaps everything that he has done was not all right. But at the moment he doesn't want to think about it anymore.

Do you believe in life after death?

No.

And now I will count to three, and then you will find yourself immediately after death. One – two – three, now you are there. How do you feel?

Well, I just feel myself very heavy. I see my body very close to me...I feel so unbelievably clumsy... I can't move properly. I can't get up....There come two funny people towards me....They are giggling and laughing....They want to take me with them....They are as bothersome as flies. They are beating me. They are kidding me. They are laughing so silly....

Where are they taking you?

Yeah,... in a big hall. Someone is standing there. A teacher,...He says something like, "You have failed completely."

Do you know him?

Yes, he is my teacher. (Here he remembers something of earlier periods in the beyond.)

What's his name?

Hieronymous.

And how do you feel, after he has said that to you?

I feel myself awfully guilty.... He says, „We'll take a long look at all that."

What occurs to you most?

My coldness, my arrogance, and my callousness - everything was just terrible. And I'm so ashamed....

Why are you ashamed?

One cannot live like that!

But as Igor you said that you had taken whatever you wanted.

But one cannot live in that way.

And what have you learned from that?

You can't take something from someone else. You have to treat other people with care.

Are you sorry for the things you've done?

Yes, but that doesn't help any.

If you were to say, "I will never again....", what would you say now?

I will never again misuse my power. I will never again force someone to do something for me against his will....For the time being I would just like to do something for others.

And what would that be?

I will probably have to return and do something to make up for what I've done.

Do you know when you will return to the earth?

Very soon.

Why so soon?

Because I'm so ashamed.

What do hope for if you return so quickly?

That I can forget what I have done... and that I can make up for it so that I can forgive myself later.

Go now to a place where you can experience how your future life will be.

It is a very light room; here they are discussing this question. There are some helpers who are discussing alternatives....They are telling me what I will be able to experience in my coming life and offering me some alternatives to choose from.

Are you allowed to voice your own wishes?

Of course!

What will you decide to do?

I will return as a woman.... I must learn to feel as a woman feels. I have to experience her strength – and at the same time her weakness.

Do you know already what you will encounter on earth?

I will be born in France.

Do you know who your parents will be?

That is still under discussion.

Have you met there, where you now are, souls who have decided to incarnate together with you?

Yes.

Who are they?

They are just soul-partners, friends.

And how will your life in France be?

I will just help people there.... I want to heal them.... I will work with herbs.

Have you ever done that?

I will learn to.

Will you learn that on earth?

No, I will learn that now.

Are there people where you are who are especially knowledgeable, who can teach you all you need to know?

Yes. Here you can learn everything.

Do those people with whom you will incarnate have some kind of special characteristics by which you will recognize each other?

They simply come, and we just recognize each other.... There are no special signs. I will recognize them in my heart.

And now Angelica is led back to the Gate of Clouds, back to her Higher Self:

Ask your Higher Self now why you had to live this life as Igor.

That just occurred. I didn't need to be so cruel in my life as Igor.

What made you actually live so cruelly as Igor?

Thirst for power, and the pleasure in seeing others crawl in the dirt. There I forgot who I really am.

Ask your Higher Self, please, if you will meet, or have met again in your present life as Angelica any of the girls you abused in your life as Igor.

Yes. One is my present husband,...another was someone I was employed by, who then really sucked me out and then threw me away.

And what about Plischka, your girl friend then? Have you met her again?

No.

Ask your Higher Self if you will have to visit another life in order to discover the cause of your present hay fever. Or are the two lives we've discovered up to now enough?

That's enough. But these two lives have repercussions in other lives.

Now Angelica is led to the Mountain of Revelation. From there she has a bird's-eye view of these two lives now spread out before her.

Do you know what karma is?

Yes.

Then why don't you compare your life as the perpetrator Igor with your life as Marianca? What effects are seen there?

They have to do with power and helplessness. Misuse of power causes helplessness. We are supposed to learn to accept our own power, our own truth, our own divine spark, which no one can extinguish, no one else can possess, which only belongs to each of us individually.

And why didn't Igor pay attention to his own inner knowledge?

He was too occupied with controlling others.

Ask your Higher Self if you had to commit offenses as Igor against your own inner truth.

Yes, I had to experience how it is to live completely in darkness. And I had to experience what misuse of power really causes.

Was it actually pre-ordained by higher powers for you to experience as Igor such misuse of power in this life?

Yes.

And were you used to balance out the karma of those you misused?

Yes. Nothing is ever in vain – the planning is perfect!

Why did you still have to suffer through that life as Marianca?

I had to experience then the opposite – the balancing out. These are all like different facets of a diamond.

Do you recognize the justice of this karmic law?

It is not even a question of justice – it is a question of existence.

Can you explain – or ask your Higher Self to explain – what that means?

All aspects of existence must be recognized and understood. There are no lower or higher aspects, and only an aspect that is experienced in life can be integrated. From the "all-nothing" [? – this word not quite clear on the tape] comes all-knowledge. We all have to go through this process.

Are these your own insights, or are you receiving them from your Higher Self?

We all know that.

Now that you are on the Mountain of Revelation do you suddenly have access to a higher consciousness?

Yes, I can see clearer now.

And now look at your life as Angelica. What has been carried over from those two previous lives into your present life? What repercussions from those two earlier lives can you see in your present life?

[The object is]... to learn, to accept one's own inner truth, to learn that no one can care for me if I don't do it myself. To learn that Love is the final source behind everything.

Why did you have to meet your second husband in your present life – he was one of the girls abused by you in your previous life?

I still had something to make good.

Are there still any repercussions from those earlier lives in your present life? Think about your hay fever....

Yes, I am afraid that I cannot protect myself.

Have your Higher Self explain what your present hay fever has to do with that earlier life.

It overcomes me. I can do nothing to prevent it. I tend then to die inside. I don't know then how to protect myself.

How do you react when you get this hay fever? Do you retreat?

I can do nothing to protect myself against the pollen. It just penetrates my body.

Are you overcome then by a feeling of helplessness?

Yes, and I feel tired. And there is itching and I am helpless to stop them [the pollen]. ...They are everywhere.

Can you see a connection between the pollen and the sperm that entered your body when you were raped as Marianca?

Yes, they're the same.... Both overpower one. One has no choice.

Are there any repercussions in your present life from the left leg that caused Igor so much suffering?

No. I just suffered from my bad nutrition habits.

This period in the beyond was to last about fifty years until the soul of Angelica was reborn in Normandy as Suzanne Bisson. Although the sense of time is relative in the so-called "beyond", Igor's soul could then prepare itself for that life as a "witch", equalizing not only a great amount of karma from the life as "Igurk", but certainly also a lot as "Igor".

But Igor's life caused a further karmic resolution - after almost 600 years - in the life as Marianca, where the source lay for her present hay fever. We can see here that this annoying condition has to do with helplessness and masculine sperm – generally in connection with rape. In this way Regression Therapy can finally offer hope in bringing effective relief to the millions of people suffering every year from this unpleasant condition.

This session is very instructive in respect to karma. It is also important for the soul to accept its own inner truth during its earthly sojourns, to express it more and more openly from life to life and finally – at the end of all incarnations - to manifest the divine spark completely and in a totally loving form in thought, speech and action.

In our subconscious we all know this. And on the Mountain of Revelation this inner knowledge and conscience often suddenly pops up again in our consciousness, for which reason clients often describe their sessions as initiation ceremonies. Thus Igor decides for reasons of higher intelligence received in the "beyond" to reincarnate as a woman, in order to experience the helplessness of a woman. After he has experienced this by being raped (e.g.), his soul will carry this on as knowledge. If then he should have the opportunity in a later incarnation as a man to take possession of a woman by force, he will remember how it feels to be raped and hold back from this desire – if it turns up again in him at all.

The country in which he is to reincarnate as a woman has already been determined, but the prospective parents are still to be chosen. He is also to be thoroughly prepared for his next life – including preparatory training in herbal medicine – so that it will be easy to re-learn this as Suzanne on earth. Everything of importance concerning forthcoming necessary experiences has been predetermined from the level of higher knowledge.

It is also important to live the life of a predator in order to experience what it means to misuse one's divine powers, i.e. one's thoughts and deeds. And it is just as important to experience the same acts that one has carried out against others also in the form of acts carried out against oneself, i.e. against one's soul. In this way the soul learns to recognize on its way through many incarnations – whether on earth, on other planets or even in other dimensions – what is the right and wrong way in its actions toward the divine unity (which is represented by the divine spark, also known as the "inner Christ") in each and every soul. All aspects of existence are to be experienced, for they belong as "facets" to this "diamond", a diamond that is to be perfected by "polishing" through the process of reincarnation.

3. When the karmic process requires several lives (Suffocation)

Robert is forty-four years old. He is allergic to pollen, especially birch pollen, and various different grasses. From April to June a swollen and constantly runny nose tortures him, tears flowing from his eyes, coughing and above all difficulty in breathing. A day before our planned session he called up to ask for an urgent emergency treatment for his terrible breathing difficulties.

After putting him into the alpha state we investigated first his present life for possible causes. At the age of three he had experienced his first traumatic loss of breath on a picnic excursion. After eating, his parents took a nap in the rather high grass while he ran around playing. Suddenly he fell down and landed with his nose directly on a dandelion flower, whose seeds flew about and landed in his nose. (*Robert coughed violently at that point in the session.*)

At the age of ten, smoke from a Bengal light got in his nose. He suddenly could no longer breathe and was also made fun of by various bystanders. At the age of sixteen a teacher hit him on the breast during boxing training, causing him to lose his breath and fall almost unconscious to the floor. In the army they trained by running with gas masks on. He could not breathe and saved himself from suffocation by sticking a finger between his gas mask and his face to let in air. These and similar occurrences were, as we would discover later, all only karmic repercussions of earlier events.

Upon being asked, his Higher Self led him into a life in

medieval Russia. He saw himself as a knight armed with a spear and a bludgeon who was just in the process of attacking a castle along with other knights. They succeeded in overrunning the castle, but in the courtyard of the castle burning tar was thrown on him and he was hit in the chest by a spear. Despite the pain, Robert perceived the stinking smell of his burning leather suit and the feeling of his burning skin. (*Robert began again to cough violently.*) While still trying to pull the spear out of his breast, he fell to the ground and died. He floated out of his body, saw how spears and burning tar hit some of his compatriots and then went directly through a tunnel into the bright light.

In his next life he is a twelve year-old boy that has to dive together with other boys for pearls. A man finds enjoyment in pushing him under water to show how strong he is. But the boy panics, and his lungs fill with water.

In another life he is a Prussian soldier named Egon who fought in 1792 against the French. While pushing a cannon he slips and falls into the mud, where one of the cannon's wheels rolls over his chest. During the attack no one can care for him, so he lies there about 15 minutes before dying.

In a still earlier life he is a five year-old native Indian boy whom his tribe has just sacrificed by throwing him into the sea to soothe the wrath of the water-god. In the beyond he meets his "predecessor", the boy sacrificed the previous year, and then floats around the world, where he is greeted with a great "Hello!" by others known to him from his tribe.

His Higher Self shows him now his life as a perpetrator as the causal life for the many oncoming lives of karmic suffering, lives in which he again and again was as short-winded as in his present one.

In one life far back in time he was a sorcerer who carried out human sacrifices by killing his victims with smoke and incantations. In a later life he belonged to the group of henchmen responsible for capturing and imprisoning women declared to be witches. His "specialty" was putting a sack over the head of the captured women, allowing them hardly enough air to breathe. After their conviction they were generally burnt at the stake. One of these women is his present, second wife.

After Robert had gone into all these earlier lives with the Golden Cup and had carried out the ritual of forgiving and being forgiven, he returned to the beta state and opened his eyes. His nose was suddenly completely free of congestion, and his coughing attacks had completely disappeared. He exclaimed joyfully, "All my problems have disappeared!"

The karmic retribution for his two earlier lives as a perpetrator had lasted many lives even down to the present one. Having recognized the reasons for his present shortness of breath and dissolved his former hardheartedness by the act of retribution, his karmic balancing process was now complete. This is a phenomenon demonstrated again and again by Regression Therapy. Therefore it seems probable that this form of therapy will "spread like wildfire". For is there anyone who does not wish himself free of annoying karma?

4. The karmic results of malicious head-wounds (Migraine headaches)

Migraine headaches are one of the torturers of mankind, especially of women (nine times more than men). We will discover the reasons for this at the end of the following case to be described.

After the synergetic therapist – let us call her "Ursula" – had discovered my book *Das große Handbuch der Reinkarnation – Heilung durch Rückführung* ("The Big Manual of Reincarnation – Healing by Regression Therapy") and had read it straight through, she called me up immediately to arrange for an appointment. Though having been successful in healing migraine in her own patients, she had suffered for many years from it herself.

Already three-quarters of an hour before the set time, she rang my doorbell. The anamnesis revealed that Ursula, the mother of two already grown sons, suffered her first attack of migraine when she was pregnant with her first son. After that she had attacks in variable intervals from one to three months, each attack lasting 3-4 days. Her whole head was afflicted, making it impossible for her to sleep, though only in the worst cases did she take medicine. Despite the fact that the migraines took away almost all of her energy, she tried nonetheless to carry on her activities, if only at a minimum level. For the past year the attacks had also been accompanied by vomiting. Among the yearlong symptoms were also constant cold feet and annoying blisters on her tongue and inside her mouth.

After she had been put into the alpha state and returned to her life as a victim, she experienced herself as Hans, a young German spy imprisoned in a Japanese prison in 1940. He was naked and freezing in the cold prison. His hands were bound behind his back and his emaciated body hung from the wall, while five men tried by various torture methods to force confessions from him. The worst of the torture methods consisted in receiving electroshocks on his feet and also in his mouth, which, as he said, drove him mad. His constant screams did not prevent his torturers from punishing his body a whole fortnight in this way, until they finally killed him by breaking his skull with iron bars. Immediately he returned to full consciousness, finding himself floating outside of his body, where he could view his decimated, bloody skull. There was immediate relief: his hands and feet felt warm again and the pain in his head had disappeared.

Led from this horrible life back to the Gate of Clouds, Ursula was informed that the Japanese man who had carried out the electroshocks and finally burst his skull with the iron bar was her present older son, with whom she had had great difficulties from the beginning and who was at that time suing her in an inheritance dispute. Now Ursula's Higher Self was asked to lead her into a life that had caused her having to experience such suffering as a German spy.

She experienced herself then as a drunken, uniformed French soldier named Pierre, who was just stomping crazily on the stomach of a fully pregnant woman. She was expecting a child from him, and he was extremely angry. Being as yet unmarried, he was enraged by the thought of the child's forcing him to marry this woman who he no longer loved, but in fact now even had begun to despise.

Before the Gate of Clouds, Ursula now learns from her Higher Self that the woman Pierre stomped to death is her present younger son, while her older son is the baby who died from his stomps. On the Mountain of Revelation the further details are revealed: Ursula remembers that her migraines began just at the time she was pregnant with the older son, the son who had also been the Japanese electroshock torturer and finally killed Egon with an iron bar. (The same son had already at an early age shown great interest in electro-physical experiments.)

Her Higher Self explains now to her that Hans had had to be tortured to death for karmic reasons stemming from the life as Pierre. The baby whom he had stomped to death had also died of a head-injury, for which reason Ursula had to suffer migraines in her present life from the iron bar injuries as Hans. Her blistered mouth and tongue stemmed finally from the electroshocks, her cold feet not only from the electroshocks but, originally, from the fact that they were used by Pierre to stomp on the stomach of the pregnant woman.

Here, as we can see, ramifications may carry over into one's present life from one's life as a perpetrator as well as from one's life as a victim. Karmic entanglements thus are subject to a strict logical process that is suddenly revealed to the client on the Mountain of Revelation – without his/her having to think much about it. Such revelations strike one suddenly and can be unreservedly and immediately accepted – one knows within that it is the truth.

After the resolution by means of the Cup of Gold, with which she asked and offered forgiveness – above all respecting her older son, whom she had killed as a fetus and by whom she had been tortured – I led her slowly via the bed of clouds and the meadow back to the waking state. She was a little dazed, which is no wonder, but she realized that something important had taken place in her life.

During the next few days she telephoned me several times with enthusiastic reports of success: "My blisters have suddenly disappeared!" Then: "My migraines are gone! I have never felt so good!" Finally: "My oldest son, who was suing me and who had stopped speaking to me long ago, suddenly relented at the court proceedings. A miracle!"

As we will see later, discordant karmic relationships are

often transformed positively by the act of retribution represented by the Golden Cup of love and forgiveness. It just happens. I could well imagine that Ursula and her older son suddenly are able to relate to each other harmoniously as mother and son. For it was subconscious rejection, or even hate, because of the fatal stomps that had led him to punish this soul so drastically as a Japanese torturer and even in this life had made him a such a rebellious youngster. Different souls recognize each other subconsciously and often begin again on the emotional or experiential level at the same place in their relationship where they had left off in an earlier life.

And now back to the question why nine times as many women have migraines as men: According to the results of Regression Therapy, Ursula's migraines, like most, originated in fatal head-injuries in one's previous life (in this case: her life as Hans). But the real cause is a life as a perpetrator, here: a life in which she killed the fetus by stomping on its head while it was in the womb. Lives as perpetrators are usually lives in which we were men causing suffering to others – often to women. To balance out such hard-hearted deeds we usually choose lives as women, just as Ursula had chosen her present life as a woman in order to suffer her second karmic balancing event in the form of migraines.

Or to formulate it in other words: Regression Therapy has shown that female migraine patients generally have received in an earlier life fatal head injuries as women. The original cause was however rooted in a life as a perpetrator in which the soul was a man who injured someone, generally a woman, fatally on the head. Regression Therapy is now revealing many previously unknown causes of illness, so that medical science must begin to accept a new way of considering the development of symptoms. Medical faculties will not be able to avoid integration of Regression Therapy into their curricula.

KARMA AND PSYCHIC SYMPTOMS

Although I divide – in agreement with modern medicine – the symptoms shown in the examples into somatic, psychosomatic or psychic types, the distinctions between them are not sharp but gradual and a strict division is seldom possible. So someone who suffers from claustrophobia may also feel a painful pressure on his/her chest, and someone with stage fright can suddenly feel a pain in his/her knee or leg before going on stage. Or someone who is afraid of speaking before a group may suffer from neck-pains before giving a public speech. Regression Therapy reveals, as we will see in the following examples, many processes that have yet to be scientifically explored – processes that over and over again turn out to be karmic in nature.

I will begin in the following examples with different kinds of fears. There is hardly anyone who is completely free of fear. But every symptom, however insignificant it may seem, must have had a cause at some time in the past, otherwise it just would not be there. Many fears have, of course, their origin in one's present life. If I was bitten by a dog in my youth, this may result later in fear of dogs - or it may not, depending on how much I took it to heart, i.e. how deeply this event has engraved itself in my psyche or my emotional body. But if we ask the Higher Self to take us back to the real cause of a canine-phobia, we will usually suddenly find the cause in an earlier life.

I remember a case in which a healing practitioner in one of my training-groups wanted to know where her fear of dogs had come from. She was afraid of even the tiniest dog. We found the cause in an earlier life in India, where she was a shepherd-boy using his club to try to defend his herd against an attack of wolves. Suddenly the pack turned and killed him. A physician who also had taken part in the session and was in possession of a German shepherd dog wanted to know if she had been completely cured and invited her after the seminar to visit him in Berlin. At the following supervision seminar she showed me exuberantly a photo in which she was hugging the dog. Her canine-phobia had disappeared as if it had never existed.

5. A boy is driven to balance his karma (Fear of deep water)

Karola is a forty year-old divorcee with one son. For the past few years she has been living with a man, Helmuth. But there are some problems in their relationship. Among all her symptoms the worst is her fear of deep water. Though she can swim, she only goes out to the point where she can still be sure of keeping her footing. She has an occasionally recurring nightmare in which a hand stretches out of the water to pull her in. So we asked her Higher Self to lead us to the life where the cause for this fear could be found.

She finds herself suddenly in France, where she is a twelve year-old girl walking in a castle recently overrun and now deserted. She lives in a neighboring village and has come here out of curiosity. There she finds three horses, that show by their whinnying that they are very thirsty. She takes a can lying there to the well to get water, but loses her balance and falls in. There is no use shouting, for no one is near. Sobbing, she tries to hold on to the slick stone walls of the deep well, but gradually she weakens and drowns in the water.

In her next life she sees herself as a five year-old boy visiting a beach hotel with his parents during the summer vacations. He feels lonely and unloved. Some power within him beckons him on to the sea so that he can go swimming with his new bathing trunks. Although he has been forbidden to go into the water alone, he sneaks out of the hotel and goes to the beach, where he puts his trunks on and enters the water, making sure that his feet are still touching the bottom. He cannot swim, but likes to feel the waves playing about him. But a wave suddenly throws him off his feet, carrying him out to sea, where he drowns.

Brought again to the Gate of Clouds, she asks her Higher Self why she had to drown in those two lives. As an answer she was taken into a still earlier life in which she was the captain of a sail-ship. Apparently there was unrest among the crew for lack of food and the captain had the leader of the mutiny thrown overboard. Despite his cries for help, they let him drown, though later the captain regretted his drastic discipline measures.

Karola learns on the Mountain of Revelation from her Higher Self that the drowned sailor is her present partner. Now it becomes clear to her why he sometimes meets her with mistrust and feels subordinate to her. Though he is certainly not her ideal mate, she has felt intuitively that she should remain true to him and not seek a replacement. Now she suddenly knows why she has to stay, for she wants to make up to him for her mistreatment of him as a captain in that earlier life.

Here we see the kind of karmic partnership considered more extensively in later chapters of this book. Helmuth has offered himself to Karola as a partner in this life to give her the opportunity to make up for her earlier misdeeds against him. And subconsciously she also acts exactly in accordance with this program - which she surely already prescribed for herself before this life in the beyond. All at once, now, she has become aware of what had been slumbering in her subconscious. She can now go with the Golden Cup to the soul of the earlier and present Helmuth and ask his forgiveness. In this way she can free herself from her responsibility toward Helmuth, her desire to take special care of him, a program that had caused her son to be jealous of Helmuth, leading to tension between the two males.

It is also notable that Karola was bothered by the nightmare described above, because dreams of that type often have to do with earlier lives. As retribution for that merciless act as a captain, she also had had to experience in two lives on her own person what it was like to drown in the water.

The five year-old boy drowned in the sea for karmic reasons. This had already been decided upon in the period of the beyond - probably the soul had even chosen this fate itself. It had not been able to forgive itself for the captain's deed. And the fateful premonition of the boy expressed itself in that irresistible desire to go into the waves alone. For, as will soon be demonstrated here again and again, fateful deaths – and not only these – are pre-established. In fact such deaths are usually pre-established by the souls concerned, in order to satisfy a compelling need for karmic balancing, a balancing that is sometimes even sensed ahead of time by the person involved. But, as we can further enquire, why is one life of retribution not enough, why does the soul have to experience two or even more such fates, one after the other? The answer is that the soul itself has to decide – in the beyond – when and how many times it wants to experience karmic retribution. If its feeling of remorse and guilt is very great, it might condemn itself to more extreme balancing, spread out over one or several lives on earth. The intensity and length of an event of karmic retribution is therefore up to the soul itself.

6. He smothered his daughter because of her speech disorder (Fear of making a fool of oneself)

In the following Regression Therapy session the client also was afraid of water – he had drowned as a ship's boy in an earlier life.

Steven was born in Greece. He is thirty years old and living for the past seven years together with his girlfriend Isabelle, with whom he often argues. Being interested in parapsychology, he says that he actually visited me to find out where he had known his girlfriend before. My question as to whether he is afraid of anything he answers in the positive. He is afraid of making a fool of himself and cannot speak before an audience of more than four people. When this fear takes hold of him, he suddenly is unable to speak certain sounds properly. He then cannot speak the 's' properly, so that 'sissy' or 'messy', for instance, become 'sishy' or 'meshy'. Even when he speaks Greek such mistakes occur. For that reason he has also visited a speech therapist, who was able to increase his self-confidence while speaking. But still occasionally this fear of making a fool of himself overcomes him and he involuntarily makes the same mistakes again.

I asked him then if we should make an attempt at

removing these speech defects as well as his fear of speaking in front of other people. He agreed right away, but wanted also to look into at least one life with Isabelle.

In the first earlier life in which a cause for his present fear of speaking in front of others was found, Steven sees himself as Emanuel, a twenty-five year-old craftsman in 18th Century France. The people make fun of him for his stuttering and his speech defects. They request him again and again to speak, just so they can laugh at him. There is now a group of young rowdies encircling him who command him to speak a few more sentences for public amusement. When he refuses, they push him. Suddenly overcome by uncontrollable rage, Emanuel tries to defend himself. Now the mob has every reason to attack him, hitting him until he lies in a bloody heap on the ground, where he dies of his wounds.

Now he experiences the exodus of his astral body while his material body is being transported into a nearby house. Suddenly his dead mother appears next to him. She approaches and hugs him. Other dead people he knows are there too. His mother leads him to a beautiful meadow in very lovely surroundings. Finally he comes upon a group of five men in white robes. One of them, apparently a bearded monk, introduces himself as Bert, his soul-guide. He answers Emanuel's question as to why he had to suffer such a cruel life with a speech defect by explaining that in an earlier life he had had a daughter with just such a speech defect who he however treated in a very rough manner.

Led back to the Gate of Clouds, we ask his Higher Self to take us into the above-mentioned life. Steven sees himself there as a wigged family man named Victor about 1680 in France. Among his children there is a twelve year-old girl with a speech defect who is obviously also mentally retarded. He despises her greatly and shows this often by shoving her away. Five years later – his wife has died in the meantime – he smothers her to death with her bed-cushion, probably hoping it will be seen as an accident. But Victor is arrested and interrogated. Finally confessing the murder of his own daughter, he is publicly hanged.

After experiencing this death, he again is met by the five men, who, without condemning him, ask what he might have done differently. Obviously he had not learned the lessons and passed the tests in connection with his daughter. He had not taken the effort to understand her in her distress and to offer her loving support. Victor now realizes his mistakes and deeply regrets his callousness. And as his guide takes him aside to ask if he is willing to make up for his malicious treatment of his daughter by experiencing similar things on his own person, Victor agrees immediately.

His guide then helps him plan his next life, in which retribution is to take place. He is to be a young man with a very noticeable speech defect, for which reason he is likewise to be killed. He will feel just as unloved, isolated and ridiculed as the daughter he has murdered. But Victor's soul is perfectly willing to accept everything necessary to make up for what he has done to his daughter.

From this therapy session we can clearly see that the subsequent retribution event is self-imposed – out of the need for drastic experiences that will prevent one's making the same hard-hearted mistakes again and again. So in most cases we choose our own karmic reactions.

Afterwards we visited another earlier life. There he experienced himself as a twelve year-old boy who, together with another boy of the same age (the present Isabelle), was doing service as a ship's boy. His unloving parents had forced this service on him against his will. Shipwrecked in a storm, they held onto a floating plank for several hours until they became faint and drowned. Certainly this was also a case of karmic retribution.

In another life Steven was a man whose wife, the present Isabelle, ran off with a new lover, leaving him behind with their common child. It seems reasonable for him to still argue with her in the present life since subconsciously he still condemns her for her earlier behavior. She, however, still remains with him despite all his accusations because she probably regrets having left him and the child in that earlier life and is trying to make up for that in the present life.

As his Higher Self revealed to him at the Gate of Clouds, Steven had had a total of four lives together with Isabelle on earth. On the Mountain of Revelation he recognizes the truth of the karmic law. Steven then takes the Golden Cup into his lives as a perpetrator and as a victim, asking for forgiveness and offering it to those involved. Then he speaks the resolution affirmation, as follows: "I free myself from my fear of speaking in front of others. I free myself of my speech defects. I free myself of my fear of deep water. And I free myself from feeling anger against my girlfriend Isabelle." Then I led him back to the present time.

It is interesting to note the following phenomenon that turned up when Victor was being questioned about his crime. When he re-experienced being interrogated about and being sentenced to hang for the murder of his daughter, his neck turned red at exactly the place where the noose must have been placed around his neck. This redness gradually disappeared, however, so that it was no longer visible on the

Mountain of Revelation.

A few days later Steven called me up, reporting triumphantly that he was now able to speak in front of a number of people without fear and, in fact, quite self-confidently. His speech disorders had also completely disappeared.

We know from therapeutic hypnosis that stuttering, lisping and other speech defects may often be eliminated, sometimes even permanently, but that they often return after some time. Thus a repetition of the hypnotic treatment may be occasionally necessary, depending on how effective the treatment – or the other way around – how resistant the programming in the subconscious of the patient is. For the client surely received at some time in his/her past a type of programming, which again may turn up in his/her present life. And even if the hypnotic re-programming does have some effect on the original self-programming, it does not mean that the latter has completely disappeared. For it may turn up again at any time when the short-term or longer term effects of hypnotic re-programming have worn off.

But if in Regression Therapy the actual root of the problem is eliminated by being revealed and forgiven, then the original self-program completely and permanently disappears.

The following example examines a further case of the fear of speaking in front of a large group.

7. The karmic reactions can be postponed but not cancelled (Fear of speaking in front of others)

Erika is about forty years of age, the mother of two school-age children. She appears to get along quite well with her husband but suffers from an inferiority complex. She sees the reason for this, among other things, in the fact that her mother had already rejected her before birth and often left her during childhood with her grandmother or in an orphanage. Erika refused to suck her mother's breast and was often beaten by her. Her mother's own marriage was terrible, her father being an alcoholic.

When she was ten, her parents divorced. Her stepfather was attracted to her and forced her from the age of fourteen until she was eighteen to carry out different sexual practices including copulation. She is afraid to speak in front of a group, not even being able to utter a few syllables at a school parents' night. In such situations she feels like there is a rope around her throat, and her throat hurts even at the thought of having to speak in front of others. While speaking even in normal conversation, she is inhibited, always searching for the right way to say something. Along with this she is afraid of authorities, whether they are the police or a court of justice before which she must appear as a witness. She is even afraid of her own husband, who is not intellectually superior to her. But somehow she feels inferior to him and always is afraid of not being able to satisfy him.

Erika suffers also from overeating. Though, as she says, she has tried all kinds of diets, her body won't get thinner. She suffers, too, from the obsessive need to agree with everyone, crying over everyone's "spilled milk" and taking everyone's suffering to heart. She only feels at ease when she can be alone and follow her own whims. She has already had numerous spontaneous reincarnation experiences while lying, e.g., under the sunray lamp. She has already starved to death while imprisoned in a tower. She was also an African warrior who abandoned his childless wife in the wilderness, abducted other women and robbed and killed many others. She was also a leader of farmers' revolts in the German Peasant's War of the 16th Century, whose throat was cut because of his "rabble-rousing speeches".

Though we discovered in the subsequent Regression Therapy session first a life as a victim and then a life in a monastery, I would like to begin with a description of her life as a perpetrator – i.e. the life that was the cause for all other karmic causal connections in her present fear of speaking in front of others.

Erika is a big landowner in Russia. His name is Mendel and he is a discontent. He controls about a thousand serfs, whom he treats quite brutally. He often takes the whip himself to chastise not only his subordinates, but also his wife and son. Whoever rebels against his arbitrary decisions faces the deadly anger of this fat little "gentleman". In other words, he is universally feared and hated. For instance, he kicks a beggar approaching him for money for treatment of his sick wife and has him thrown out.

At the age of sixty he is poisoned. He does not know whose work it was, but with his last words he curses everyone. Once outside of the body, he sees how jubilant everyone is over his death. Now his wife takes control, and because he can now read thoughts he realizes that she had poisoned him. From the conversations of those still living he realizes what a devil in human form he was. Now he is gradually beginning to feel ashamed and sorry for many of his misdeeds.

Suddenly he finds himself in darkness. He meets some persons who were, like him, very malicious on earth but who have already begun to regret their acts. From advanced beings visiting them in this realm of darkness – into which more light is now gradually entering – he learns that he and the others in this area have actually acted against their own best interests: they now will have to experience the same suffering that they have caused to others.

Mende is ready to make up for everything and to experience himself all those misdeeds that he has carried out against others. One of the teachers suggests that he could best go through several lives in which he can prepare himself for a life of karmic balancing. Among others, a life as a nun was suggested, in which he could learn humility and modesty to moderate his explosive temper. Mendel agrees immediately to this suggestion, as he hopes as a nun finally to learn to love and to atone for his many sins.

Before the Gate of Clouds Erika learns that the beggar Mendel drove away with kicks is her present brother and his wife her father, who had abused her sexually as a girl. This relationship is strongly karma-laden and will possibly be the subject of another Regression Therapy session needed to clear it up completely.

About a hundred years later she is a nun, Maria, wearing a black hood under vow of silence in a French monastery. She was brought here at a young age after the death of her parents. Here she was forbidden to speak, even to other children. The only kinds of speech allowed were prayers, or answers to the questions of the strict but fair Mother Superior. She was told again and again that one should have no desires of any kind. Maria finds this atmosphere stifling and from day to day she suffers more, finally confessing to the Mother Superior her desire to leave the monastery. She is told that this is no longer possible because she has made a vow before God to remain there forever as His humble servant.

Maria is now torn inwardly by the dilemma whether to follow this order or that of her own heart telling her to leave the monastery. In her prayer to God and to Jesus she thinks she hears an answer telling her to follow the call of her heart. But upon stating her final decision to leave the monastery she is told by the Mother Superior that God now damns her for breaking her vow. She then leaves the monastery on foot. It was, like she now says, like a grave for her.

Then she took a job as a maidservant on a farm, where she later married a farm-worker, had a daughter and enjoyed, as she now says, a pleasant life until she died at sixty. Before the Gate of Clouds she hears from her Higher Self that the previous Mother Superior is now her own mother, who, as we remember, wanted nothing to do with her, sending her whenever possible to a children's home or her grandmother's, or beating her whenever she was at home. Subconsciously her mother was still angry with her for leaving the monastery as Maria in her earlier life.

We humans would be much more tolerant and understanding toward each other if the following facts were always clear to us: Everyone's behavior is based on previous constellations, i.e. on programming. If we ourselves were subject to the same experiences or programming as someone else, we would act just as he/she does. We human beings must free ourselves at last from our ignorance - or worse: from our refusal to acknowledge things that we actually already know. Then we could live more consciously and responsibly. The author of this book would feel great pleasure in being able to make even a small contribution toward this goal.

It was to take more than 300 years until the actual karmic

rebalancing for Mendel's misdeeds could take place. Certainly there were other lives in the meantime containing karmic balancing events for Erika's soul. But it was not possible to uncover them all in this one session.

In the final karmic balancing life Erika experienced herself as a thirty-six year-old craftsman in the German state Sachsen in the year 1570. His name is Johann Pilscher. He is married, has a child and owns a small house near the entrance of a small town. At this moment the people have assembled on the town square, angry at the heavy taxes leveled by the ruler of the state. Those who are not able or willing to pay, have been beaten or imprisoned. They choose Johann to carry their complaints to the ruler.

When his wife hears of this decision, she knees before him and begs him not to go along to the palace. But Johann is determined not to change his decision to represent the others. A group of about fifty men now approach the iron gate of the castle, demanding to speak with the ruling sovereign about the oppressive taxation. The ruler, however, is not willing to speak to them, but sends a messenger to tell them to go home or he will have them driven there by force. The following dialog develops, which Johann now relates:

"We cannot pay anymore."

"Hold your tongues!"

"We cannot pay anymore....There must be changes made. ...We will not leave until we speak with the Prince."

The guards ridicule the craftsmen, to which Johann responds by striking through the gate after one or the other of the guardsmen. But they have already sent for militia, who now come, have the gate opened from inside and then attack the rebellious townsmen with all the weapons they have with them. Johann's throat is cut. He dies immediately. Now he floats over the whole scene, returns with the others to the town and is present when his wife is told of his death. His wife begins to cry, and so does Johann (i.e. Erika; *for such cases I always keep paper handkerchiefs ready!*). And then he sobs, "I shouldn't have done it."

When I give him the cue: "I will never again...", he completes the sentence: "...hurt my wife. I should have listened to her." Later he visits his wife again as a ghost, watching as she re-marries. *Often it is the passed-away partners who arrange new marriage-partners for their spouses.* For karmic reasons, Johann had to experience how his wife was mourning in great desperation, for he himself as Mendel had driven so many to such outbursts of mourning, anger or desperation. If experiencing his wife's tears had not been necessary for his karmic training, he possibly would have been led back into the beyond immediately after death.

Erika called me up already on the same day to tell me joyfully of her great relief at experiencing a totally different – more relaxed – perspective. So we can see that everything is planned down to the smallest detail in order to lead us to greater and greater abundance of love. And, as we have also seen, karmic balancing for an act need not always take place in the following life, but may be postponed for some lives while other things are taken care of. Sooner or later, however, they will have to be cleared up: karmic reactions always catch up with us – unless we are so advanced that we can fully clear the account on our own. But we will deal with this possibility later on in the present book.

And I am sure that she will soon realize that she can talk to groups without any fear. For this fear was generated in the life as Johann for he was killed because of his bold talk and acting. This fear Erika stuffed into the pine cone and thus was released from it.

8. When karmic connections are carried over for centuries (Fear of standing in front of the public)

Veronika is a thirty-year old concert pianist, who suffers from rye pollen allergy and sneezes constantly from May to August. She has to earn her living as a piano teacher because of – and that is her real problem – her fear of the public. She can always play her pieces perfectly while practicing them at home, but the nearer the concert comes the more her fear of failure and disgrace grows. She always walks the floor nervously even weeks before her planned concerts, and hours before the concert she is so preoccupied that no one can speak to her. When she finally sits in front of the piano and starts to play, she is dogged by the fear of playing the wrong notes. This often causes her to make mistakes even in relatively simple pieces such as Mozart's Sonata KV 330. For this reason she now prefers only to accompany singers, though the singers often are infected by her nervousness, too. Though she is single and could easily change professions, she feels an inner need to play piano in public.

In ancient Rome she was once a corrupt and bribable judge who could put such pressure on an accused person by clever rhetoric that, even though he was known to the judge to be innocent, the accused would become unsure and contradict himself. Accepting false-guilts as true, he even stooped to bearing false witness himself against the accused in order to convict him and bring about his execution. But later his conscience bothered him so much that even before his death he swore, "I will never again bear false witness!"

In accordance with the law of karma and as a result of this life as a judge, Veronika's soul had to experience similar acts against itself for several further lives. Her Higher Self led her into two of these balancing lives. In one of them she was a German politician in the 19th Century who in rhetorical battles with opponents – in spite of his political commitment and his other talents – became insecure and confused in his arguments and, instead of establishing his position, usually ended up losing the debate. Thus he hurt not only his own reputation but also that of his party. Sooner or later he was asked not to give any more speeches, at which point his political career was ended. In that life he had to experience on karmic grounds a part of what had been experienced by those persons he had falsely accused and convicted earlier as a judge.

The balancing of malicious karmic burdens goes its own complicated way. Surely Veronika's soul had had to balance out many other things in the many centuries between that life as a judge in Rome and that as a German politician and very probably had itself been wrongly condemned to death at least once. The reason why her Higher Self did not lead Veronika into such a life but rather into that of the German politician was because we wanted to uncover why Veronika made such mistakes in her public music recitals.

In the next life to be unraveled she was a German pianist named Isabella Polditz, born in Cologne in 1903. She had a similar fear of public performances, suffering public disgrace on account of playing mistakes before finally resigning herself to life as a music teacher in Hamburg. Thus the helplessness and insecurity of the persons accused and convicted by the Roman judge had to be experienced in at least three lives by Veronika's soul in order for it to understand what it means to be made unsure and to suffer from stage-fright.

We can see that the law of karma has a "long arm", reaching from callous deeds committed centuries – or even more than a millennium – ago into the present, to force us to balance our karma out. And all of the – large or small – problems that we experience in our lives most probably belong to that "autodidactic" karmic curriculum of the soul. Thus now there are possibly thousands of different threads from earlier existences, many of them having karmic connections, all woven together to make up the fabric of our present life-situation.

A year later Veronika got another appointment for a Regression Therapy session because she wanted to finally rid herself of her disturbing pollen allergy. On arriving she announced joyfully that she had lost all her fear of playing in public and that the singers she accompanied were now surprised at her strong nerves. She even said that she had played with great success at the state competition for Brandenburg and in a national competition in Cologne.

How many hundreds, if not thousands, of stage performers suffering from stage-fright could finally be freed from these disturbing side-effects of karmic entanglements and would no longer need to turn to alcohol to control their fear? Of course, if they are forced to keep on suffering from stage fright for karmic reasons, then even Regression Therapy will be powerless. But what can they lose by making the attempt?

9. The karma of a Roman soldier that ended in his present life (Agoraphobia)

Martin is thirty-seven and very friendly, though somewhat shy. He suffers from a bad case of agoraphobia, which sometimes even becomes claustrophobia. He is afraid of big crowded places. A full stadium would be a nightmare for him. A crowded train, tram or bus is like hell to him. In such situations he cannot even swallow and has to gasp for air. Especially threatening and frightening is the presence of any number of men! in an assembly where men are present he can hardly get a word out.

Martin was easy to put into the alpha state, but on the Bed of Clouds he began to breathe heavily and showed all the signs of being possessed by a ghost. Now I spoke to the ghost and even got it to speak. The ghost was a construction worker named Hans Meyer, born in Bale (Switzerland) in 1923, who said that he had made a mess of his life. He hated women, in fact all people – including himself. Finally he had hung himself in his own house. He had first entered Martin when he was weakened as a child with the mumps and had remained since. We were finally able to successfully free them both. Hans' dead mother then came to lead him to the beyond.[35]

The question arises here whether possession by ghosts is itself connected with karmic balancing events or not. For someone who at present is possessed by a ghost could have been in earlier times himself a ghost possessing someone else – who he then depleted of energy, drove to irresponsible acts or even controlled with his will. In fact possessed persons often feel themselves weak or caged-in, and I suspect that there may indeed be a karmic connection. Certainly we will soon have more details concerning this question.

We then asked Martin's Higher Self to lead him into the

---

35. I refer those interested in the question of possession by ghosts to Edith Fiore, *The Unquiet spirit,* and Carl Wickland, *Thirty years among the Dead.*

earlier lives connected with his agoraphobia. To present the case in a more logical way I will begin my description with the life as a perpetrator again, including verbatim some parts of the dialogue from the tape:

Martin experiences himself as a Roman centurion who has about 1000 soldiers under his command. He is wearing breast armor and a helmet, is forty years old and calls himself Geani. They are just in the process of attacking a large town in Germany.

I will now count to three. Then you will experience yourself carrying out an important act. One, two, three. What are you doing now?

We are just attacking and killing the people.

What orders do you give your soldiers?

To make everyone unable to fight. My only interest is making them incapable of defending themselves. Nothing else interests me.

And how do your soldiers carry out this order?

They steal, rape, and kill - children, too.

Where are the men of this town?

They are very well equipped to fight.

Why was it necessary to plunder, rape and also kill the helpless?

Yes, that's the life of a soldier....One becomes callous.

And you are there, too, and you kill, too?

Yes.

Is there a special experience there for you?

There is a monk there with a brown robe....He curses me.... And I am astounded that he has so much courage...Now I want to see how much courage he has....I ride on my horse up to him....Yes, he stands fast....Somehow I know that he is right. But I have my work to do.

And what do you do with him?

With my sword I cut his head off with one blow.

Does anything else of importance happen?

No. But somehow this incidence has moved me. For he made no move to retreat, though he knew that I would kill him.

Are many people in this town still alive?

Yes.

What happens to these people?

We rest a few days, then we move on. We kill all the men, and the women have to cook for us.

What happens to the children who are still alive?

They stay with the old people.

Asked to go on with the description of his life and his misdeeds, Geani describes how he is involved as a high-ranking officer in Greece in major battles and finally returns to Rome. He dies there at the age of sixty-nine as a wealthy and politically influential man from poison given to him by a servant as the result of a political plot. I ask him if he has any regrets at the end of his life. "No, I was satisfied with my life. But so much of it was just a waste of time."

Asked the usual key sentence, he answers, "I will never again be responsible for the death of so many people. But most of all I mean my own people. The others are not so important." Arriving in front of the Gate of Clouds and his Higher Self, he learns that what he has done was important for him – he just had to do it.

Why did you have to be the commander and cause others so much suffering?

To learn that power can also be misused. Having already killed so many people, I could have said that there was no use in that and just retired from the scene.

Here the Higher Self himself indicates clearly that to school ourselves as souls in proper thinking and acting we must also at some time involve ourselves in guilt and even abuse our power. Reflecting on this abuse, we can then learn to refrain from it in future lives. Every abuse of power – necessarily involving hard-heartedness because it entails injury or suffering for others – must be balanced out for oneself by experiencing helplessness and injury at the hands of others. We are involved in abuse of power in order to learn never to do so. The only purpose of the law of karma is to make us feel on our own body or soul what we have caused to others as a result of our own callousness and abuse of power. Everything occurs according to a great plan. Considered from this vantage point, there is actually no guilt, because we are purposely entangled in guilt.

The perceptive reader will have noticed that many lives as a perpetrator took place in Roman times, when the Roman Empire was being expanded with the greatest brutality in all directions. And for some reason many of the balancing lives as a victim took place in France – as in the following case, in which we will see how the law of karma was fulfilled for Geani:

Martin is now a woman of twenty-eight at the beginning of the 17th century. She found it so boring in her village that she left at the age of eighteen for the city of Nancy. However, finding no work, she is forced to sleep with men and finally lands as a prostitute calling herself Felicitas. She and her fellow prostitutes are subject to the ridicule and contempt of the Catholic population. For obvious reasons they are protected by the military stationed there. But when an important official accuses her of picking his pocket in a tavern, this protective hand is withdrawn. The common people claim she is in allegiance with the devil, and she is condemned to death by decapitation. A clerk reads the written judgment to her in her cell.

Experience now the day of your execution. Where does it take place?

On a large square.

Are there many people there?

Yes. But I'm not the only one to be executed on this day.

Who else is there?

There's a man there too, a murderer.

Where are you now?

Next to the platform....Three soldiers are holding me. I have to wait.

What do you feel now?

I am afraid, but somehow I am also not afraid.

Do you despise the people there?

Sure.

Are they screaming something at you?

They are screaming, "la pute", the whore.

Describe now very exactly your last three minutes. What is happening?

They are bringing me up there....I have to lean over...They are binding me fast.

And what is to be used for your execution?

An axe.

Who takes the axe?

A man, who has a hood on, so he can't be seen. (We remember that Geani cut off the head of a hooded monk.)

And now I will count to three. You will find yourself outside of the body. One, two, three....How do you feel now?...Can you see your cut-off head and your body?

Yes.

Is the murderer still there, is he still being executed?

No, he was executed before me.

How does the crowd react? What kind of feeling do you have for the people there?

Somehow it is a triumph for me because I am still living....I feel much better now than before.

And if you said one sentence beginning with, "I will never again...", what would it be?

I never want to have anything to do with men...I will never move again without preparation to a town where no one knows me...I will never again trust city people. I have seen how the people in this city really are.

And now I will count to three, and you will experience your most wonderful experience after your death. One, two, three. Where are you now?

On a meadow,...flowers,...trees. Everything is so peaceful.

Are you alone there, or is anyone else there?

No, there are only children. I am responsible for them. ...And I feel very good.

What do you like best there?

I am glad to be together with these children.

Why are you attracted to the children?

Because they are honest....And because I have actually always wanted to have children.

Surely the reader, too, is pleased to know that, after a life in which we have experienced a drastic karma-balancing event, we are allowed a special experience of the pleasures of life in the beyond, particularly being blessed with the joys of what we had most longed for in our previous life!

I now led Martin to the Gate of Clouds and requested

him to ask his Higher Self why he had to experience such an awful death.

What does your Higher Self say?

I had taken on a lot of guilt before. I didn't treat people so well. ...It was in my earlier life.

But before we entered the life as a perpetrator (already described above) in which the soul of Martin had experienced or caused the guilt for the now balanced deeds, I requested him to ask his Higher Self whether there was another life in which a further reason might be found for his excessive fear of the public or of men. So his Higher Self led him to a life as a low-ranking Prussian officer named Alfred:

I have about 30 men under me....It is in the country, over there are the buildings we live in.

What is happening there?

We are practicing....We are preparing for something...to receive some important guests...

I will count to three, and then you will experience an important event for you. One, two, three. What is happening?

The soldiers have something against me....They have prepared something....They are standing at a certain place.... Now the important officials are there. And I have to command my soldiers....And suddenly they throw cow-dung on me. And everyone watches....I slip and fall. Everyone laughs....And the important people see it too. They laugh, too.

How do you feel, when they all laugh?

They have made a fool of me.

And your own soldiers have done that to you?

Yes.

And what do you do?

I run away....to my own quarters....I cry....I hang myself.

What do you feel after death?

I am sorry for what I have done.

Do others come? If yes, what do they say?

They are very shocked.

Are you happy that they now feel remorse.

I see now what I have done wrong.

And I will count to three, and you will experience your most wonderful experience after death. One, two, three. What do you experience?

There are many other soldiers who I knew, but who had already died. They are all very open and warmhearted. They take me like I am.

And what do they say to you?

That I am welcome here.

What are you most surprised about?

That there are no rank differences here.... We are all equal, no one is superior.

Do you believe that they all know what has happened to you?

Yes.

And no one laughs?

No....They are all friendly.

After you had hanged yourself and died, did you come here right away, or what did you do?

No, I waited there at first to see what would happen. When they saw me hanging there, they called the others. But then the beings from the other world, they came and took me.

Who took you?

They were some of my own soldiers I had lost in battles.

If you were to say now, "I will never again....", what would you say?

I will never again have control over other people....I often stayed back myself and sent my soldiers into battle.

And that was why your soldiers didn't like you?

Yes....I never want to be in the military again.

Now I led Martin to the Gate of Clouds back to his Higher Self.

Ask your Higher Self what you were supposed to learn in that life.

I should have taken over responsibility and shown courage.

This was a test for the soul that had taken on Alfred's body, a test whether it would again be misled to become an unmercifully ambitious soldier of Geani's type or whether it had learned to avoid killing. And obviously this soul had learned in the many centuries between that of the Roman centurion and that as Alfred the Prussian soldier to avoid needless killing. Thus Alfred's alleged cowardice was possibly more a product of such a self-programming as: "I will never again kill." This soul had made great advances since that life as a Roman soldier.

Another interesting fact made evident in Regression Therapy is that a life as a prostitute is generally also based on karmic reasons. Here there are usually several preceding lives as a perpetrator in which the soul has been a rapist. A prostitute's life is usually chosen by the soul, on the one hand, to punish oneself for what it had done to women before. On the other hand – and primarily – it wishes to have an experience of being humiliated similar to what it had caused earlier to others.

10. When different phobias are connected with one another (Fear of heights, fear of snakes, fear of speaking in front of other people.)

Jennifer was born 52 years ago in the heart of Africa, but came to Europe already at the age of eight. She is now married for the second time and has a daughter from her previous marriage. For a long time she worked in the fashion line, but is now a Reiki teacher. She has numerous phobias and other symptoms: fear of being deserted, of success and/or failure, of speaking in front of others, fear of heights and snakes as well as hay fever, smoke allergy and myoma with part extirpation.

Many persons in Europe share the fear of snakes. But because they seldom come in contact with them, this symptom may remain latent until a suitable situation arises in some successive life. Because Jennifer lived as a child in Africa, she had the opportunity to see several snakes and is thus became aware of her phobia. But first we asked her Higher Self to lead Jennifer into the earlier life where her fear of speaking in front of other people is anchored.

She experienced herself as a 30 year-old Greek orator in the year 403 B.C. His name is Anatolio(s), and he stems from a well-to-do family. She sees him dressed in a white toga, surrounded by numerous disciples, with whom he also occasionally is sexually intimate. One of his favorites is Kostas, the son of a politician in the present government who was very angry at Anatolio for misguiding his son and for holding public speeches apparently aimed at unseating the ruling party. This' father has now managed to get Anatolio arrested and condemned to death for agitation of the youths. He is then executed by being thrown into the water from a high cliff.

When I asked him what he would never want to do or experience again, he said, "I will never again speak in front of groups in public." This life also contained at least one of the sources of Jennifer's fear of heights.

In the next life relevant to Jennifer's fear of speaking in front of people she found herself suddenly in the body of a 40 year-old Egyptian slave named Assan. Previously he had been a farmer who criticized corruption in the state too openly. His neighbor, who was in love with the same girl and jealous of Assan's success with her, had denounced him in the hope of eliminating his rival. His rival's plan being successful, Assan was soon sent to the stone quarries, where he had to work twenty years with chains on his arms and feet, often suffering, too, under the whips of the guards, until he finally lay down exhausted and died.

After the question before the Gate of Clouds about another life connected to his fear of speaking, Jennifer saw herself as a ten year-old French boy named Claude at the turn of the 19th century, who was born dumb, so that he was later unable to speak. He became ill and died at fifty.

Arriving again at the Gate of Clouds, Jennifer learns the names of some of the people from her previous lives in her present life. Then she is taken into that life that is the cause for all those lives suffered as a victim. There she experiences herself as an African princess named Kina, who is engaged to a prince from another major tribe. Kina has great influence on her father, who as the ruler likes to follow the advice of his darling. She is, despite her young age of 23, of a very evil mind, considering lies and intrigues as only the least of her instruments. She appears quite inventive in her methods of eliminating her enemies: some are thrown from the cliffs to the crocodiles, others are beheaded. A priest speaking unpleasant truths about her had his tongue cut out after being accused of lying.

At the age of forty, with six children, she takes over the reign from her father. But she is hated by the people, and, finally, at the age of forty-five, one of the co-wives kills her by putting a poisonous snake in her bed. And the lives described above were only three of the many resulting lives as a victim in which she had to experience retribution in quite different ways for her deeds as Kina.

It is interesting to note that her life as a perpetrator was lived in a female body. For in most lives as a perpetrator we see males, who as a result of their physical strength - combined with ego and ambition – commit aggression against women and others. From my experience I would calculate that about 95% of all of the more aggressive lives as a perpetrator are lived as men, who then experience about 60-70% of their karmic balancing lives as women. Kina, the female perpetrator, is shown on the contrary in three male lives as a victim.

At the Gate of Clouds Jennifer hears from her Higher Self that her husband from her life as Kina is her present first ex-husband while the priest whose tongue she had cut out is her present partner. Here we have a good example of having to meet again and again with all those souls who we have mistreated in any way until we are able to make up in a loving way for our offenses.

And Jennifer has this chance in her present life. If she can make up for all her previous offenses by treating her present partner with love and respect, then there will be no further need to meet again for karmic reasons in future lives. Their present meeting in this life was certainly already decided upon in the preceding period in the beyond. Her present partner was willing to give her the opportunity to finally eliminate her offenses as Kina against him. It is also interesting to note that Jennifer's soul did not clear up her guilt for cutting out the priest's tongue – thus making him "speechless" – until her just previous life. We remember that Claude was already dumb ("speechless") at birth. The time difference between Kina and Claude may have been over three thousand years. So we can see that time is often of no great consequence in karmic rebalancing.

Three of her many symptoms were uncovered in previous lives and could now all be rebalanced. This is one of the phenomena characteristic of Regression Therapy, namely that while uncovering one symptom other symptoms from other lives are discovered. These symptoms can often be simultaneously resolved by putting them also into the pine cone – i.e. on the condition that these symptoms do not require the opening of other lives for their resolution. But we can gain more information in each individual case from the Higher Self.

11. When birth is a karmic event (Fear of closeness)

Ulli is a psychotherapist who has become well known through his books. He is about 50 years old and suffering from a special type of claustrophobia: fear of tight places. He became very aware of this while taking part in an Indian sweathouse ceremony in America. The Red Indian was sitting very close together with about ten people in a small igloo-type hut covered with branches, blankets and skins. In the middle was a small pit filled with glowing hot stones on which sage-water was poured. The steam-filled air then caused the half-naked men to sweat in the dark hut while singing ritual songs.

These sweathouse ceremonies have a religious and also a therapeutic purpose, namely to rid the body of whatever does not belong to it, e.g. ghosts, negative thoughts or magic curses. But Ulli suddenly panicked. Gasping for air, he shoved the doorway blanket aside and left the hut. It was hours before he could calm himself down again.

Something similar had already happened to him in the Osho-ashram in Poona, India. In an "experience-seminar" thirty more or less naked participants knotted themselves into one great human knot. Then Ulli was also overcome by panic and, wildly flailing with his arms, he escaped from the mass "knot" and fled from the room. He was overcome by similar anxiety when being held by others in a group therapy session. In a spontaneous deja-vu experience brought about by a similar case of panic, he had suddenly seen himself as a village idiot being grabbed by ruffians and held under water until he drowned.

We experience often in Regression Therapy that claustrophobic patients get stuck in the birth-channel during birth, where their chest is compressed, causing near-suffocation. When he told me his father died three weeks before his very difficult birth, I decided to take Ulli back to the time when he was a fetus.

Going as a soul into the fetus at two months, he sees that he is to have a twin brother. The latter's soul, however, never enters the body. Thus the dead second fetus is rejected by the mother's body in the fourth month. Ulli is already afraid as a fetus, as he senses it will be a difficult birth. He experiences in his eighth month the thoughts and words of his mother when visiting her dying husband and hears his father screaming at her. When his father dies three weeks before his birth, he then feels his mother cramp with grief.

There are no accidental events whatsoever in creation, so these experiences of the fetus must also be seen as karmic events. He was supposed to experience the feelings of his mother because he had – as we will soon see – killed the husbands of many women, among which many were surely pregnant. Their children experienced also the sorrow of their mothers and, of course, grew up without fathers, having to live with all the disadvantages of such a childhood.

His own birth in the hospital is traumatic. Although his head was in the right direction, his body refused to go through the birth channel. The doctors had to yank him out forcefully by grasping his head.

At this point I have to explain some things in order to make karmic birth events understandable. If a soul has had to live trough the terrible experience of being buried alive or squeezed in – events that are often fatal – and if this experience has imprinted itself on the emotional body, then the emotional body will repeatedly create states of panic whenever there is a stifling situation. Therefore the fetus can also experience a normal birth as traumatic when it has to pass through the birth channel. When, however, a soul traumatized by such pre-conditioning has a difficult birth, then it experiences real panic.

However, this experience of panic by the soul is just part of the well-planned karmic dramaturgy. And it was for this reason that after two months in the womb Ulli's soul was afraid in advance of what it was in for. The soul in the fetus still usually remembers the karmic events already planned for the coming birth. And a difficult birth belongs to such plans.

It is therefore understandable when many well-informed

people say, "Everything is karma", thinking not only of bad but also of all the good things which a soul experiences. But this version is certainly not correct. I would formulate it differently: "All experiences have a purpose; nothing happens by chance. Everything serves the purpose of our becoming loving persons." But, whether they are good or bad, most of the events experienced by a soul arise from the interaction of cause and effect..

Ulli sees himself now as a higher-ranking English soldier named Fopar, about 40 years of age, at a feast of King Henry, whose subject and liegeman he was. Fopar seems to be his lord's expert on gathering young peasant girls by force for such feasts, where they are made excessive sport of. Fopar's parents were killed by a predecessor of the present king when he was five, but he himself was still brought up at court and enjoys now this privileged position.

In the next scene we experience him during an attack on a village. It turns into a bloody battle in which he takes full part with his sword. Everything living there is killed, except the women, to which the soldiers – intoxicated by victory - now turn. But at the age of 43 his fate turns against him: during a battle against King Richard he is struck in the breast by a lance while sitting on his horse.

In the next life - as a victim - Ulli was a prostitute named Miriam, living in Asia at the end of the 15th century. She lived in a hut, where she was also visited by her men customers. Because of her beauty she had been educated as a temple prostitute and was considered as worthy of special worship, being under the protection of the priests. But one day a drunken man comes to her hut. When she refuses his wishes, he becomes angry and tries to take her by force. She takes a dagger and screams at him, saying, "If you come near I will stab you!" When he continues his attack, she stabs him in the neck.

Others hear his cries and rush into the hut. Seeing what has happened, they hold her down. When soldiers lead her off, her rival prostitutes stand in the crowd, screaming hateful words. They are glad that their rival – preferred by the men because of her beauty – is now out of the way. But Miriam makes no effort to resist as she is taken to prison. The city magistrate condemns her to death by stoning.

On the day of her execution she is taken in rags outside the city gates, where about a hundred persons have assembled to enjoy this spectacle, among them also several men casting sad glances in her direction. But Miriam has been in a state of shock all the time. She is bound to a stake. A soldier makes a short speech. And now many of the bystanders, among them women, take up stones and throw them at the bound woman. When she seems to be dead, they take off the ropes, lay her body on the ground and cover it with the stones thrown at her, adding earth for good measure. But Miriam is not quite dead. She comes back to consciousness under the stones, sees the soil being thrown over her and experiences now death by suffocation.

The reader will now surely understand that this is the reason why the soul in the body of Ulli is later struck by fear of closeness. And in his attack of panic in the sweathouse stones were also visible. Thus Ulli's fear of closeness is a repercussion from the victim's life as Miriam, which was chosen on karmic grounds as a part-consequence of her life as a perpetrator as Fopar. This fear of closeness is therefore a karmic reaction.

But Miriam's experience continues after death. She sees

herself naked on a silk-covered bed. She feels completely healed of her wounds. Beings in white robes come and stroke her and smile to her. She does not know what has happened in the meantime since her death. She goes in a transparent dress through a wonderful garden. She can eat and drink, but somehow her experience is different, not material as she is accustomed from the earth. She meets a man who looks like a prince. He kisses her. They gaze into each other's eyes, and she feels an indescribable eroticism in her whole body. It all seems like a fairy-tale. But one should realize that in the beyond one can transform imagination into reality, which is then lived as such. If one is not capable of this upon arrival there, others may be helpful by producing such reality and allowing one to take part in it.

Asking Ulli's Higher Self which of the persons in that life as Miriam have reappeared in his present life, he hears that he has already encountered some of the prostitutes from that life or still will encounter them. But Ulli learns even more. His soul was supposed to experience the bad side of Fopar, his callousness, in order to learn how one feels when love is missing in one's life. His hard-heartedness, by which many were caused to suffer in body and soul, had to be balanced in a number of later lives as a victim. The life as Miriam was only one of these, but it was the one we were looking for, the one responsible for his fear of closeness.

Furthermore Ulli learned that he had had up to now about 900 lives as a perpetrator and about 1500 lives as a victim. And many of those lives included both of them. For we must consider that in many lives we carry out things injuring others and at the same time we ourselves also experience suffering. Lives as perpetrators and lives as a victim are intertwined in many ways. We know, for example, that many criminals had a hard life as youths, being beaten, suppressed or even abused, thus having to balance out karma before they could perpetrate karmic misdeeds again. These callous misdeeds then help others to balance out as victims their own karmic reactions.

In my seven-color novel MOLAR, covering the karmic events in Germany's most bitter time during the Second World War, I name such persons "wheel-rotator" because they keep the wheel of karma in motion. They allow others to balance their karmic burdens by helping them to experience suffering as victims, while the perpetrators add karma to their own burdens, only to be relieved of it again through intervention of still other karmic perpetrators. Karma perpetrators and karma balancers thus condition each other mutually.

But let us now turn to claustrophobia itself in order to investigate its hidden karmic causalities.

12. When one has buried others alive in another life (Claustrophobia)

Liane is a single woman in her middle thirties. She suffers from depressions and loneliness. Besides a pollen allergy she also suffers from difficulty in breathing or sometimes even asthma, which began already in her youth. She also has a fear of heights, keeping her from going up sightseeing towers or flying in airplanes. And besides a fear of spiders she also suffers from a grave case of claustrophobia that kept her already as a child from riding in elevators.

All of these symptoms are warning signals for the karma researcher, for here karmic reaction patterns are obviously at work. They offer us deep insights into previous lives as a victim and thus also into lives as a perpetrator. In this case we began with the breathing problems, but soon discovered that claustrophobia was closely connected to them, so that eventually both problems could be cleared up.

Suddenly she finds herself in southern France at the beginning of the 13th century. Her name is Esklamadura, and she is the wife of a count. They both belong to the Catharians, a sect that has broken with Rome and is now being persecuted by the Catholic Church. They have already experienced a great deal of suffering in their lives. She sees the murdering hired bands of the Church torture, massacre and burn all the Catharians whenever they find them. All of the houses of the Catharians are burnt down. During a siege of their own castle, in which she loses several children and sees parts of the castle burn, she chokes and is almost suffocated.

Considered to be one of the leaders of the sect, she is able at the age of seventy-five to escape to the last bastion of the Catharians, Montségur Castle. This castle is on a steep mountain and is considered invincible. But soon this castle too is encircled by the army of the Church and begins to burn from the many fire projectiles. Esklamadura suffers again from choking attacks. And as the enemy is near to overrunning the castle and she falls unconscious, she is put in a partly covered stone casket to keep her from being discovered. Still able to breathe, she eventually regains consciousness and tries several times unsuccessfully to push the plate off. In the meantime the enemy has taken over the castle and burnt many of the Catherians at the stake in front of the castle. Undiscovered and still conscious, she lies there three days while smoke from the burning wooden beams keeps entering her casket. Then she loses consciousness and dies.

She now floats over the destroyed castle, then over the surrounding land - everywhere there is destruction! Then she is, as she says, "pulled into the light". This light cures her of all her ills. She sees the members of her family, her relatives and friends, who all have died in this Christian war against the heretics. They are wearing white robes. She meets there a wise man, who explains to her that she had to experience all this suffering because it is a part of the universal plan. All beings, whether man or animal, wish to suffer, which is a part of their freedom. When Esklamadura rejects this statement, the wise man says that she will just have to accept it for the present. Suffering is the pre-condition for all development: one loves in the same way one suffers - love is learned by suffering. (Negative) Karma is the result of wanting to suffer. For we have all chosen this suffering in order to attain love.

I have only copied down the wise man's words, conscious of the fact that they are still unordered. And I can imagine that many readers want to protest against them, and from their standpoint they are right. Anyone on earth who publishes such words will be considered crazy. But in the last section of this book we will take another look at these statements from a higher standpoint and perhaps modify our opinion.

When we asked her Higher Self if there were not any other lives in which a cause for her present breathing difficulties could be found, Liane was led into a life in ancient Egypt. She was an eighteen year-old priest named Siris. He had just secretly entered a strictly forbidden room said to be a place where one could see the gods – at the immediate cost, however, of one's life. Curious, Siris risks it all the same and is surprised that he is not immediately struck down. Though inside there is total darkness, he has a vision of a being calling itself an "unknown god". Instead of wanting to be worshipped itself, it actually only desires to make men to gods. Thus the "god" considers itself Siris' brother. But the priests are afraid, it says, of losing their own power if men no longer worshipped the gods.

When Siris leaves the forbidden room still alive, several young priests bow down to him in wonder. They think the gods must have spared this courageous young man because he is perhaps also divine. But the older priests put him under arrest. He is subjected to herbal steam mixed with poison, making him completely lame. Still conscious, his body is then mummified – except for mouth and nose - painted gold and placed in a sarcophagus, where a death mask is put on him and a living poisonous snake laid on his body. Then the sarcophagus is closed with a stone plate and shoved into an opening in the temple wall. Siris remains a long time in this immobile state, still breathing while the snake lies next to him.

After a while Siris does leave the sarcophagus in his astral body, but to his horror he discovers that he cannot leave the Anubis temple because the priests have imprisoned him here with a magic spell. After some years or centuries the Anubis cult is dissolved, and a new cult uses this temple. Reading on the sarcophagus that the "sleeping youth" is contained there who saw God and spoke with Him, they start a cult in his honor. To occupy himself Siris finds in the temple a priest being psychic through whom he – being able to read the minds of the inquiring visitors – speaks exact oracles.1200 years later, after the spell of the Anubis priests has lost its effect, Siris is finally able to leave the temple.

As Liane now hears from her Higher Self, she was next reborn in the year 214 A.D. in Persia. Furthermore she is told that the cause for both of these lives in which she was incarcerated in a stone casket was the fact that she had also had persons buried alive in an earlier life. Her claustrophobia is a karmic result of both these lives as a victim, and ultimately of that life as a perpetrator.

Her depressions and loneliness, as the Higher Self continued to explain, stemmed from the long years in the temple but also had other karmic reasons. Her pollen allergy came among other things from the poisonous herbal steam that was used before mummification. Her difficulty in breathing came from choking and finally dying as a result of smoke asphyxiation in her life as Esklamadura. For karmic reasons it was not yet possible to be totally free of these symptoms, though a considerable improvement is going to take place.

So in the resolution affirmation Liane was able to free herself from her pollen allergy, her claustrophobia, her loneliness, her difficulties in breathing and – as always in such affirmations – from all of the guilt feelings still present from her life as a perpetrator.

It is interesting to note, that for some cases the Higher Self states, that there can not be a

complete release of all symptoms because the unwinding karma has not come to its end yet. But if further on asked if there could be gained at least an improvement, the answer will be in the positive. And this applied as well to Liane. For after this session some of her symptoms were declining or even stopped completely.

13. Even knowing and ignoring can cause karmic reactions (Fear of sexuality)

Johanna is a thirty-eight year-old civil servant. She has never been married but is living with a partner with whom there has been no sexual contact for the past eight years. Johanna is extremely afraid of being raped, though in this life nothing of this kind has occurred. She is afraid of the woods because a man could be waiting there to attack her. She is also afraid of pregnancy. At eighteen she started taking the anti-baby pill "just in case", though she had no contact with men. At fourteen years of age, when her menstruation began, it was accompanied by strong cramps. For the next four years these cramps reappeared every menstrual period.

Johanna now sees herself as Brigitte, the daughter of an influential aristocratic father at the middle of the 16th century in France. At twenty-three she would certainly have been a good match in higher circles in her golden shoes and long white and gold dress if her character had paralleled her appearance. But she is arrogant and impossible to please.

She has a cool relationship to her father. Her mother is no longer living in her father's palace at the edge of a forest, where Brigitte loves to ride out with men, outdistance them in horse-races and to play with their hearts in society. She is careful not to let them come too close.

At the edge of the forest one day she sees a girl with torn clothes pleading for help. The men had stopped in the forest to avoid riding by this girl. Brigitte knows immediately what has happened, for she knows well the rapacious desires of some of the men in her company. It is clearly not the first time that she has made aware of the callousness of her companions. She knows that she herself has made these men rapacious by her own coquette behavior. Laughing, she only mocks the girl and rides on.

But her conscience tells her then that she should have stopped to help the girl. The sight of the girl occupies her thoughts constantly. Out of disgust for men she never marries. When she is asked after death what she would say about her life, she says, "I will never again be heartless."

But, as we shall see, this callousness was to have karmic repercussions in a later life. For not only our active deeds produce karma but also the things we fail to do – out of indolence, disinterest or malice. Her mocking smile was already a sign of hardheartedness. Every act of callousness, even if only in thoughts or words, requires karmic balancing – as a subsequent life of Brigitte will prove.

The soul of Brigitte was reborn in the Bavarian Forest around 1770 as Maria Pfeiffer. Her father was a forest worker and her mother already dead when we meet Maria, at the age of 15. She was walking in the woods, collecting cranberries with a basket under her arm. Suddenly three men turned up, encircled her smirkingly and began pushing the mortally frightened girl with their hands. Her basket fell to the ground. Then they threw her on the ground, tore open her blouse and pulled her skirt up....Only two of them violate her – the youngest is too afraid or feels sorry for her. Finally they leave the girl and go their way. Her blouse is torn, her skirt full of cranberry stains, and blood is flowing down her legs.

With shaky steps she walks home, her only wish being to die. When her father demands, "What has happened to you!", Maria starts to cry, moaning, "Something terrible has happened." After hearing the whole story he asks her if she recognized any of them, which she denies. Taking his rifle her father starts to go. Maria, fearing the worst, tries to stop him, but he storms out into the forest.

I take her to a year later, to see if she has a child. She says no. But I had the feeling that something terrible might have happened. Had the father killed the child after birth to protect his daughter from the shame of an illegitimate child? At any rate she would not go into it any further, so I turned to another track. For one of the commandments of a regression therapist is that he always respects the free will of his client, even if the client is experiencing an earlier life at the moment. As she said, she thought constantly of this terrible experience of being raped. Also she felt so ashamed in front of her father, who was the only one who knew the whole story. Nevertheless she never developed a closer relationship to him.

I led her to the time one day before her death. She was thirty-nine. She had never married and was still living in the same house. Her body was very weak. Having spent all her energy, she grieved over her wasted life.

After death she meets her father, who treats her very lovingly. She meets other souls wearing purple-colored robes. She feels as if a terrible weight has been taken from her shoulders. A group of five souls is caring for her. She admires a waterfall that she sees there crashing down over a cliff and wonders why the cliff looks transparent.

I expect from my past experience that this life as Maria must have been preceded by one or more lives in which she as a man committed rape. But apparently her Higher Self was not prepared to reveal those lives because Maria was not ready to take a look at them. The Higher Self knows what it can reveal to a soul and what not. One will therefore never discover more than one is able to stand. Therefore no one need fear that he/she will be confronted with things exceeding the soul's ability to accept them. But, in any case, every horrible life must be therapeutically resolved immediately, before the client can be sent home.

This case demonstrates quite clearly that even passive heartless behavior brings about karmic reactions forcing a soul eventually to undergo drastic learning processes. But let us turn now to a totally different type of fear.

14. A cardinal acquires karma (Obsession with washing oneself)

A regression therapist who was once a trainee of mine called me up, asking if I could possibly come her way some time. She had taken on an exceptionally dramatic case that she did not trust herself to treat. A man about forty years of age had an unusually compulsive need to wash his hands. He was distraught and had often considered suicide. The case was urgent. She lived about five hundred miles away, but luckily I was to give a seminar nearby the following week, so I could come by afterwards.

The same day I met Rudi. He was very intelligent and creative. Himself a medium, he carried out spiritual healing on others. He was even able to see the inner organs of others by laying his hands on their bodies. He was an only child. His mother had died years ago, but she still accompanied him invisibly, offering him advice whenever needed. Rudi had certainly had Platonic relationships with women now and then, but had never carried out sexual intercourse with men or women.

After finishing his military service as a draftee, he happened to see a film in TV on the topic "The Living

Skin". Mites and blackheads were shown. Bacteria, spores and viruses living on the skin were described. While seeing it for a second time on videotape, he suddenly began to itch! Soon he was itching all over his body. This led him to scratch, and soon scales began to develop, above all in the genital area, behind his ears and on his head. And parallel to this there was a compulsion to wash himself, an occupation often taking hours at a time.

Whatever he touched had to be cleaned again with water or cleanser. If he touched the door-handle without cleaning his hands beforehand, it would have to be carefully cleaned again. If he touched the toilet bowl with his trousers, then he would carefully clean his trousers with alcoholic cleansing liquid. Of course he let no one into his apartment because the visitor could be infected with his germs. Here we can already see why he had no intimate relationships. Later we will discover still another reason.

He could not leave the house in the morning without showering at least once. Once there was no water all day because of a broken pipe. Although Rudi had an important appointment, he could not leave the house, not being able to shower beforehand. Because of his lack of bodily contact he was lonely, even though through his work he met many people. This threw him into periods of deep depression worsened by a guilt complex of unknown origin. He could not remember any significant incident in this life in which he could have acquired this degree of guilt. I myself was also curious as to the karmic reasons leading to this combination of exaggerated hygiene and dandruff. For everything that turns up in the present as a symptom must have been caused at some time in the past. Modern psychology would have seen the cause for his over-cleanliness in his strict, dominating father. But the real causes lie, as regression therapists have come to recognize, much deeper.

Dear Reader! After having experienced now so many investigations into the hidden causes of present symptoms, do you perhaps have an idea where dandruff in connection with compulsive washing could originate? Please consider this question a moment, before you read on!

Now Rudi sees himself as a thirty year-old man dressed in robe-like white and red garments. The year is 1782, and he calls himself Jean Paul. (*His actual name was Latin:* Johannes Paulus, *but in Regression Therapy sessions the names of earlier lives are often translated into one's native language.*) He comes from an aristocratic family and is already a cardinal at his relatively young age. In this function he is now overlooking the preparations in the Cathedral of Toulouse for the birthday celebrations of the king. I was, of course, curious, so I asked him a few things about his private life.

Following the family tradition he joined the clergy at the age of seventeen with the aim of becoming a cardinal. Before this he had only slept with three women, although he felt no attraction for homosexuality. His hobby was archery, and he liked to take part in archery competitions.

I ask him to go to the next important event in his life. He sees himself standing next to the high altar in his precious clerical garments, while the bishop celebrates mass in front of a packed church. Now suddenly a procession of monks in habits enters down the red-carpeted center aisle. In their center they guard a man in chains, recognized by Jean Paul as his father, the Viscount of Cherbourg. He is accused of heresy. A clergyman steps forward and accuses the Viscount of freethinking, because he opposes the

Church. Jean Paul's feelings are now divided. He was never able to stand his father. Should he use his influence to try to save him or let him be condemned and executed? I ask him if there are other reasons making it inadvisable to aid him. He confesses that he himself is also under observation by the Church, as he is suspected of having a secret love life. If he now tries to help his father, it could cost him his cardinal's position. Later, before his father is to be executed, his mother pleads with him to undertake whatever is necessary to save his father. But the son refuses on the grounds that there is no way he can help in this case.

After the death of his father he is constantly bothered by his bad conscience. I ask him if there are additional reasons for his bad conscience. He says, "Yes." When he was five, his seven year-old sister drowned before his eyes. She screamed at him to throw the big ball they were playing with into the water so she could hold onto it. But he failed to do this and has had a guilty conscience about it from that day.

It is understandable that I would like to know more about where the feelings of guilt in his present life originated. Perhaps they were all coming from that life. Sensing that he was still hiding things from the life as a cardinal, I asked him if there was anything to those rumors about his love life. Gradually he admitted it. But I wanted to know more, so, after I promised to maintain secrecy, he confessed to having occasionally secret affairs with women, and even having caught venereal disease at the age of twenty-five, from which his penis and other parts of his body were inflamed and afflicted with pus. It was very painful for him to urinate, but he was afraid to seek medical help because it would mean losing his cardinal's hat, possibly even being totally disgraced.

And soon a rash had spread to his feet and hands. He began to wear gloves, letting no one into his private rooms, especially not his bedroom, for fear that someone could see the wounds on his skin. If it were discovered that he had these well-known signs of venereal disease on his body, it could be seen as God's punishment, proving that he could no longer be His servant. Therefore all these telltale markings had to be kept hidden by means of powder, tape, very long shirt-arms and gloves. He let his hair grow longer to hide any noticeable signs on his neck. But the illness was spreading out more and more now, with rashes on his chest and elbows.

And when I asked him if that was the reason he had never again touched a woman, he confessed that, although he knew the danger of infection, he had discovered an eighteen year-old girl picking apples who had readily surrendered to him. When I enquired further, it turned out that he had in fact taken her against her will!

We see that also in Regression Therapy sessions souls may try to hide things. But sometimes it is still possible to talk them into surrendering important information. *As a regression therapist one develops gradually an intuition – despite our respect for their privacy – as to whether things are still being held back that the souls would actually like to confess.*

It was clear to him that he would infect her. But his anger about his illness and the blame he put on the women made him ignore in his sexual need all other considerations. And when he was asked if he was not afraid of God's punishment, he confessed actually not to be very pious. And when he was asked if this incident had had any further consequences for the girl – whose name was Hélène – or for him, he reported as follows: Hélène must have noticed during this act of rape his infected places, for she went to the bishop and told him about the rape and his infection. Jean Paul was taken before a church tribunal and forced to undergo medical examination. The secret was now out, and he was given the alternative of accepting the judgment of the Church or being denounced. Jean Paul accepted the clerical judgment, which meant degradation to the level of bishop without a post. The whole thing was to be kept a church secret. Hélène was recommended to join a monastery and told to keep quiet about the whole thing. Dying at the age of eighty-three, Jean Paul's last statement was, "I never want to be put to shame again. I will never again have sexual contact."

Before the Gate of Clouds, Rudi hears that Jean Paul's father is his own present father. Now it becomes clear why the two had to meet each other again and why his father is so strict and reproachful, causing Rudi to feel his guilt-complex and depression even more keenly. For, as we will see, one is forced again and again to meet certain other souls until an unresolved earlier relationship can be harmonized or forgiven in another life.

In this case we learn from the Higher Self that we have still not discovered all the causes in this session but that from five to seven more earlier lives will have to be investigated in order to clear up all his problems. Nevertheless this life as a cardinal was the most important step in the development of his syndrome. Its discovery made possible the resolution of eighty percent of his problems.

Now I would like to ask the reader again: Would you,

dear reader, have guessed what karmic causes existed for Rudi's compulsive washing and his skin problems? Hardly! As a regression therapist one is repeatedly confronted with new revelations. One is like an explorer, a Livingstone, Amundson, Marco Polo or Sven Hedin, constantly discovering new countries – in this case on the psychic globe of mankind. And how many new countries are there yet to discover, yes, even new continents unsuspected by science.

As we have seen, Rudi's life as a cardinal is in many ways affected by karma. His self-programming leading him never to have sexual intercourse is still having an effect on his present life. The skin-rash and the inexplicable feelings of guilt toward his father, which he still has to bear in his present life, are repercussions of his actions then, and his present activities as a "wonder-healer" come from a need to make up for his previous misdeeds. His obsessive need to wash himself is conditioned by his previous attempts to hide his guilt as a cardinal.

However, the further investigation and resolution of other lives as requested by his Higher Self I left up to another regression therapist. When I called Rudi three weeks later, he reported that the therapy had not yet been completed, but that to his surprise he already had regained his self-confidence: "I have become a different person. The self-confidence which I have been lacking for more than ten years has returned." The compulsion to wash himself had decreased. My colleague had also freed him of the possessing earthbound spirit causing his depressions.

What a boon it is, what a benefit for all mankind, that we now have Regression Therapy - at least for those who want and are allowed to take advantage of it because the time for them to be freed from their karmic burdens has come!

15. The body as a karmic map (Fear of knives)

Viviane is thirty-one years old. She is shortsighted and also has a fear of heights preventing her from looking down from any house or high cliff. There is a mole behind her left ear, an inch in diameter with a black spot in the middle. Her whole body is also covered with birthmarks – her face, arms, chest, and her sides down to the thighs. One of her worst handicaps is her fear of knives. She can hardly take one in her hand, and if she tries to cut meat with one, she begins to shiver, finally dropping the knife.

It was not easy to put Viviane in the alpha-state – it took three attempts. We started with the fear of heights. Her Higher Self led her first into a life in which she was a 14 year-old orphan living with a mother of twins. The woman, however, did not hide her dislike of the girl, whose depressions then drove her to jump from a cliff. She watched as a fisherman drug her body from the water, was there during the funeral and recognized her stepmother's satisfaction over not having to care for her anymore. Then she saw a woman in black laying a bouquet on her grave – this was her real mother, who had been unmarried and thus forced to give away her child. She followed her mother home and experienced her husband beating her.

Before the Gate of Clouds she heard from her Higher Self that that mother was also her present mother, her present grandmother the previous stepmother. To the question if there was any other life necessary to clear up Viviane's fear of heights her Higher Self answered that no other life was of consequence in this connection.

As this had gone very quickly, we went on. I decided to then attack the knife-phobia and requested her Higher Self to lead Viviane now to the cause of this phobia.

She is now suddenly a bank-clerk named Edwin in the year 1894 in Germany. 35, he has a girl friend named Isabelle, who is also – secretly – being courted by his friend Paul. Isabelle and Edwin decide to marry. When Paul hears this he is obsessed with the idea of murdering Edwin. He breaks into Edwin's apartment, waiting for him to return. When Edwin returned Paul stabs him with a knife in the head. Edwin, dying immediately and being instantly out of his body still sees Paul wipe off the knife and put it away. I ask Edwin how he would answer if he had to say, "I will never…." He says, "I will never be injured again." *Now the entranced Viviane begins to cry.* "I don't trust people. They are two-faced."

Edwin is also at his own funeral. There he sees his girl, but behind her stands Paul. No one has suspected him yet of the murder, not even Isabelle. Edwin, as a spirit, tries now to protect the helpless Isabelle from Paul.

How do you do that?

I don't know, it doesn't work.

Does she surrender to Paul?

No, she commits suicide.

After death they are united again. Going back to the Gate of Clouds, Viviane learns that Isabelle is her present boyfriend, Urs, and Paul is her present uncle. Then I ask her to ask her Higher Self, who presents itself to her as a visible angel, why she had to experience that brutal death as Edwin.

What does your angel say?

I was myself bad once. I killed a lot of people.

And then we asked the angel to lead her into that life.

Viviane was in the body of a fifty-four year-old, fat, black-bearded Viking, wearing a kind of helmet on his head, from which two cow-horns stuck out. His name was Hanbel (*or maybe Hanibel*) and had a long sword in one hand while he carried a round wooden shield covered with nail-points. He had already killed numerous people, plundered and, of course, raped whenever he could.

Do you have any enemies against whom you fight?

No, no enemies, I was an evil man.

How many people have you killed already in your life?

Many.

Did that give you a good feeling?

Yes. (*Said with satisfaction and pride. Perpetrators act generally in Regression Therapy sessions like real scoundrels and generally show no regrets. Only perhaps toward the end or afterwards do these appear.*)

What kind of reputation has your behavior brought you?

They are all afraid of me.

Do you do all those things alone or in a group.

Sometimes with a group. But alone it's better because I don't have to split the booty.

He is notorious, and the people in Norway and Sweden are afraid of him. It is the year 1249. A year later he falls into a net stretched over a hole to catch him. The "monster" has finally been caught and cannot free himself, so the people come and shoot arrows at him. He is covered with arrows now and, seeing himself from above, he looks like a hedgehog. From the Higher Self we hear that he will have to experience now three lives as a victim to make up for this life as a monster. Furthermore we hear that the many birthmarks on Viviane's body exactly mark the places where the arrows entered his body. And, truly, as we could discover later, we can see from the position of the birthmarks on her body exactly in what position he must have lain in the net while being hit with the arrows from above. So we went on to look at the two remaining lives:

In the next life of karmic retribution he is a four year-old boy named Michael (*spoken with an English accent*). His parents are farmers in America. They have to move and look for a new place to live and farm. They are both sitting in the front driving a wagon pulled by horses. It is night.

I sit in the back....Play with the dog....Sit on our things....I fall out of the wagon....Fall on a stone....Hurt my face....My jaw hurts.

And how do your parents react?

Drive on....The dog barks....Parents don't hear. Wagon too loud.

Can't you call?

No, I can't.

What happens after that?

I keep lying.

Don't your parents come?

Yes. They find me in the dark....I am not living....I still lie there. It is so cold.

Can you see despite the dark what your parents do?

My parents are completely dejected.

And how do you feel?

I was only playing. Then I fell out.

Is there someone there to pick you up?

No, only my parents are there. They pack me in a woolen blanket. My mother holds me in her arms and cries.

These experiences after death belong to the karmic balancing event – he has to experience as a child how parents feel when their child has died. He had occasionally killed as Hanbel sons and daughters or taken the most precious possessions away from people.

In the next life Viviane is a young Red Indian girl of sixteen. She is called Cher Wina, which means, as she says, "Light Cloud". She is alone in the forest, but secretly observed by a white man.

And now you know what happens.

He comes from behind a tree. He attacks me....I 'm not able to move away....He grabs me....He treats me badly....He rapes me.

And I will count to three, then you will know what has happened. One, two, three.

I am still lying on the ground....The man has left....I am not living any longer.

What did this man do to you? Did he knife you?

No. He broke my neck. I was screaming. He pushed my head back.

So you have died. What else happens?

I am with my mother. She knows that something has happened to me....She knows for sure that she has to look for me...They find me and take me home.

The men try now to find the traces of the murderer, but he apparently could reach safety already.

On the Mountain of Revelation we learn more details from her angel about the karmic relationships between her earlier lives. The life as the Viking perpetrator Hanbel required only three lives as a victim to make up for his misdeeds. But in his own life – namely at his death – Hanbel had had to experience a karmic balancing event, so that we can speak of four karmic balancing events in all. He did not have to experience a life as a raped woman for each of those raped by him, but was only raped once, experiencing a violent end as a raped Red Indian girl.

The intensity of this experience may have been great enough to implant in the soul a strong enough feeling of horror, so that the wish would never come up again in a later masculine incarnation to rape a woman met alone in the forest or elsewhere. Every misdeed experienced on our own body forcing itself deep enough into our emotional body will keep us from repeating such a callous act against someone else. The intensity of the event in a life as a victim is decisive for the amount of balanced karma. Thus it is not a question of quantity but of quality.

Nevertheless, there is still free will. A soul may condemn itself during a period in the beyond to karmic balancing by saying, e.g., "I have raped so many women in earlier lives. I at least need to be raped several dozen times in order to punish myself for my past misdeeds and also to feel how it is to be raped, so that I never do such a thing again." Out of its own free will it may set the amount and distribution of karmic punishment by saying, e.g., "I would like to be raped in three lives as a woman three times each." For one's free will has priority in planning a coming reincarnation, although consultants may point out different consequences and alternative possibilities.

I request her to ask her angel where her shortsightedness comes from. And the prompt answer is "Fear of life....Fear of too short a life." When I ask her if she means the two short lives as Cher Wina and Michael, she confirms.

Now ask your angel where your nail biting comes from.

I can't protect myself then....I don't want to hurt

people....I can't hit people, I can't hit animals....I don't want to hurt anyone anymore. That has to do with Hanbel.

This is certainly a completely new diagnosis of fingernail biting. For as Hanbel she had hurt people. Subconsciously she now wants to protect herself from ever being a perpetrator or an attacker again. So even nail biting can be the consequence of a life as a perpetrator.

Furthermore Viviane learns that the mole behind her ear is a repercussion of the fatal wound that she received as Edwin from Paul. Such marks serve as reminders of previous events. And we have the possibility today by means of Regression Therapy to discover these events in other lives. It seems possible to me that as a result of balancing such birthmarks may disappear in time, as their purpose as reminders has disappeared. But there must be more research in this direction. In any case, it can be said that birthmarks always point to events from other lives, unless they happen to be caused in the prenatal period by injuries. Thus birthmarks on the body may be seen as maps of earlier events that are still to be investigated.

KARMA AND SOMATIC SYMPTOMS

Somatic symptoms are those that pertain wholly or essentially to the physical aspects of man. Because many somatic symptoms are paired with psychic ones, there are even among traditional medical practitioners those who think that so-called "classical somatic syndromes" are actually 90% or even 95% of psychosomatic origin. For instance, a stomach cancer has usually to do with problems and stress, kidney problems have to do with problems in one's love relationships, leg-pains express that one is afraid to go where one should, back-pains have to do with uprightness, migraine with sexuality and problems with one's mother etc. Thanks to Regression Therapy we are able to see that even all somatic illnesses – even broken bones – originate in problems of the soul. For there is no possibility of breaking one's leg or losing one's arm in a car crash "by accident". Everything has its reasons. And where there is a deep-seated reason, there must be information saved in the mind or the soul which allows it to become manifest.

In the following examples from my experiences in Regression Therapy I would like to describe a small selection of somatic symptoms, beginning with the head and leading downward finally to the feet. Let us begin then with headaches.

16. When karma goes to one's head (Headaches)

The brain is the "grand central station" and at the same time the "end of the line" of all trains in local and long-distance "nerve-traffic". Therefore there are a great number of very different types of headaches coming from the different parts of the body. And the pains registered there can affect the whole brain or only parts of it. They may be long lasting, momentary or also cyclical. There are headaches of a constant or a changeable nature, of an aching, pulsing, hammering, stabbing nature etc. And sources in different parts of the body may signal to the head, "Something is wrong here." Thus illnesses of the kidneys, the liver, the back, the stomach, the abdomen, the neck, the blood, the skin or the sexual organs etc., or, muscle tension, nerve irritation, disturbances of the metabolism or the immune system as well as many other things may be the source of head-aches. There are even sources in the parts of the head, such as teeth, ears, eyes, nose, maxillary sinuses etc. In addition there are many psychosomatic as well as psychic origins for headaches (for instance headaches stemming from anxiety, such as fear of taking a test) and also those that may be traced back to change of altitude, weather changes, ecological influences, so that hundreds, if not thousands, of causes may come in question for headaches.

Monika is a single healing practitioner of thirty-one, who finished my course as a regression therapist. I have seldom seen anyone who had so many psychic, psychosomatic and somatic symptoms at once. And in these training courses she has been freed from most of them, either by myself or by one of the other trainees. Just to name a few of the symptoms: fear of heights, nightmares (with black men's hands grasping her around the neck), epileptic attacks (even collapses, three times even *grand mal*), asthma and throat tightness, thyroid-gland based weight-problems, a whole array of different allergies – from hay fever, mold, cleansing-powder, nickel, chrome allergies down to a wide range of allergies against different fragrances. Furthermore she suffered from a reading phobia, fear of falling, of failure and many other fears. She was burdened by depressions, suffered from an inferiority complex and massive guilt-complexes of an unknown origin. She also had a helper syndrome. The anamnesis list would have to be extended almost infinitely to include all the other fears, problems and other symptoms that she carried around with her! Hard to imagine how much time and trouble physicians and psychotherapists would have had to invest to help her overcome all those problems! If they even had a chance using their methods to alleviate all of these problems effectively. But her most disturbing problem was the constant headaches – an assortment of the most varied kinds.

They began when she was a child. Sometimes they were in back of the left eye; sometimes they attacked the whole head. Sometimes they were short-lived, sometimes they lasted for days. Sometimes they were accompanied with nausea and/or vomiting. An eye-migraine was diagnosed. Her sensitivity to perfumes, cigarettes, and exhaust-gases was often the trigger for spontaneous headaches. Often her headaches were combined with back-pains or are caused by tension in the neck. At the age of nine she fell over backwards and hit her neck on a jutting edge, etc. etc. For the headaches alone her anamnesis would have to be much longer.

I demonstrated Regression Therapy on Monika to other seminar participants, leading her first into her life as a victim. But to facilitate understanding of her case I would prefer to start with her life as a perpetrator.

Monika sees herself as a thirty year-old Roman soldier over-running at the moment a village with about a hundred other soldiers. This succeeds by unimaginable slaughter. His name is Petrus and he is something like the worst of the commando troop. He commands a prisoner to take a few steps and then whacks his head off from behind, only because he has bet with his comrades whether the prisoner would take a few more steps or not before he falls over. And he wins the bet because the prisoner actually does take a few more steps. The others laugh or clap their hands. Petrus enjoys his role, showing off his brutality to others. At thirty-five he plays another dangerous rogues' trick: He boards a ship secretly and cuts the three watch-guards' throats, stealing jewels and other valuables. His comrades praise him, and he says proudly, "No one can beat me." Murdering, drinking, whoring, raping, stealing belong to the everyday activities of his "hero's life". At forty-two he finds himself in a tavern gambling for money. Everyone has to let him win, or risk losing his life. He makes a special joke of animating new guests to play and then, when they think they have won, to kill them in front of the others, saying, "See, I am the winner after all."

When he is about fifty, he gets stabbed in the abdomen in a fight. Stumbling back to his room, he bleeds to death there all alone. And when I ask him if he regrets anything, he answers, "I regret nothing." In real scoundrel manner he is even proud of his deeds and claims, when I ask, to have killed about fifty people out of pure mischief, whether by stabbing, beating, strangling, neck-breaking or in whatever way possible, not even counting all those killed in battle.

He wanted fame and power. That he had obtained, without a doubt. But at what price? For whatever he did to others, he had to experience on his own person according to the law of karma. If he had recognized the validity of this law then, would he not have relented from his criminal deeds immediately? The worse the suffering one causes for others, the worse one's own fate will be later, including all the repercussions down to the present day. If we spoke before about the birthmarks being a karmic map, now we can add that the total diagnosis of the patient's illnesses represents the inner map of his/her karmic past.

From the many karmic lives as a victim resulting from this one scoundrel's life, Monika's Higher Self chose three that – because this was our starting point – were connected with headaches.

She sees herself as a fifteen year-old acrobat in Italy of the 16th century, who is traveling with a group of artists, three brothers and their friend, from one place to another to perform their sometimes foolhardy stunts in public. His name is Martino and his act is to walk a tightrope while manipulating rings with his hands. Suddenly overcome with fear, he stands as if paralyzed on the platform above. He signals to his comrades that he cannot go on. But they call to him, saying he should hurry up and go on. His knees now begin to shake. One of the brothers climbs up and practically pushes him onto the tightrope. From below the curious crowd peers at him high above. There is no net to catch him. When he reaches the middle of the rope, his knees begin to shake more. He falls, his head hits the paving-stones and he dies immediately. After death he finds himself in a kind of fog. Suddenly shining beings in a golden light approach him. Their smiles are visible, but not their whole faces. One of them takes him by the hand and leads him into the light. Arriving in a room full of light, he discovers other entities in a white light. They all seem to be transparent.

In another karma-balancing life he is a seven year-old shepherd boy named Michael in the Alps. It is 1920. He is sitting on the fence of the family enclosure. His father has left to get the other sons. A cow is about to calve, and the other sons are supposed watch the event in order to learn how to help. Michael climbs into the enclosure alone, despite having been forbidden to do so. He touches several cows, then notices that the cow is already giving birth. He moves closer to help in case the birth should be difficult, just as he has seen his father do. While he bends down, the cows are frightened by the approaching cries of his older brother and his father for him to come out immediately. Michael is knocked over by the moving cows and his head, back and whole body got hit by the hooves of the cows. He dies from the injuries. His last "never-again" sentence: "I will never be too self-confident. I will never attempt anything on my own again." (*Monika had, of course, brought a fear of cows with her into her present life.*)

In the next life opened by her Higher Self, Monika was a fifty-four year-old woman named Margit living with her four year younger husband, Peter. Although he is not an alcoholic, he hits her often to prove his dominance over her. She is afraid of him. His anger has also to do with the fact that she has borne him no children. Once, when she was pregnant, he kicked her in the stomach, causing a miscarriage. But Peter blames her for this. Peter is unemployed. It is 1951, and they live in a village in Germany.

One day as she is coming down the stairs, Peter is sitting in the kitchen, waiting for his meal. He curses her, "You are good for nothing, you ugly cow." She feels worthless and is also ashamed. He gets angrier and angrier. He stands up, grabs her pigtail and shakes it, then pulls it and slaps her in the face. He tears her dress, letting her breasts show. She is ashamed. The choleric man hits her head now against a wooden post, keeping on and on until she has the feeling her head will burst. She still sees his angry face, then her skull breaks. She dies. Suddenly she stands next to her body, that despite the flowing blood is still being hammered against the post. She feels no physical pain any longer, but she is still suffering psychic pain. Finally Peter lets go of her, her body then falling to the ground.

I ask Margit what she would say if she began, "I will never again…" She says, "I will never again meet someone who is so evil. I will never again be beaten." Finally she floats over a beautiful meadow. She has now arrived in the beyond.

At the Gate of Clouds we hear from her Higher Self that she should have left her partner and not let herself be humiliated. And when I ask about the causes for her present headaches, her Higher Self says that a total of seventeen lives have been determining factors for her present headaches. As an answer to another question of mine we learn that we now do not have to visit any of these further lives. So the headaches should be over now.

And in fact after this Regression Therapy session all her headaches disappeared never to return. A year later she reaffirmed this, saying that through the Regression Therapy carried out by me and the other participants she had become a totally new person, full of energy and zest for life. Her inferiority complex was gone together with her guilt feelings; there was no sign left of back pains. She said she had never felt as good before. As a non-medical practitioner she had been already specializing in back and head problems and with the addition of Regression Therapy she was able to treat many more patients successfully.

I knew that Monika had a helper-syndrome. She was always ready to help anyone who needed help, especially if they had physical problems. A helper syndrome is a subconscious expression of karmic guilt feelings from the fact that one has injured persons in earlier lives and has the wish to help now where ever help is needed. This is the reason that many people with a helper syndrome take up medical professions or work in life counseling, social welfare or care of old people etc., where they have sufficient possibilities to help people. If they help others gladly, not unwillingly, they will be in a good position to work off their karmic burden successfully.

And in the medical or social professions one will specialize in that area in that one has injured others the most and therefore where the greatest karmic guilt exists. That is why Monika had specialized in back and head problems, those areas in which she had suffered most up to the time she began her training in Regression Therapy. In many instances one does not become a heart surgeon, gynecologist, mid-wife, urologist, nurse, kindergarten teacher etc. by chance but because one is drawn to that area in which one (subconsciously) has some karmic debt to repay. Of course, this choice is already made in the beyond, where one already begins to prepare oneself.

So it was not necessary to investigate all the lives connected with Monika's karmic headaches in order to cure her. But this raises the question again: Why does one person have to suffer through only one life as a victim to achieve karmic balance, whereas another has to suffer two or three, still another five or more lives as a victim? This depends on many factors, not only on our voluntary decision in the beyond. Above all, it depends on the intensity with which we experience a balancing life. The soul can experience e.g. being raped in different ways: by leaving the gross body and evading the experience altogether, "coping-out" by becoming paralyzed with fear, by subconsciously affirming the experience out of guilt or by experiencing every moment of the rape as a terrible, shattering attack on one's person. To repeat again, not the number of evil deeds perpetrated in a villain's life is to be equalized in the lives as a victim, but the intensity of the acts is to be balanced by the intensity of suffering.

17. Karmic reactions can occur on different continents (Tintinnitus)

In respect to number of symptoms Eberhard can even outdo Monika. Some of them have already been a puzzle for medical science. For almost everything possible is there: depressions, inferiority complex, fears, allergies, heart-muscle disturbances (five months in the hospital), headaches, migraines (with vomiting), feeling of tightness, bronchitis, asthma, fear of people, fear of being disappointed, claustrophobia (he cannot enter elevators), hemophilia (periods in hospital), neck and back problems, tinnitus and dizziness (also with psychiatric treatment). His chin is often out of joint, he has an alcohol phobia, he has a number of problems with his mother etc. etc. etc. And we have hardly mentioned half of the problems. So karma is back in play!

As a child he was already putting on girls' clothes and his obvious homosexuality was a great source of ridicule during his childhood. Later he even had problems developing relationships with men because of his fearfulness and various complexes. So for a long time he had an unfulfilled sex-life. Military service was painful for him, and if there had not been nice men's bodies for him to view, it would have been intolerable. It seemed strange that he could even have been drafted.

A few months before I had freed him from fear of heights and bridges. Now he could cross bridges again. In a supervision seminar I chose four diploma candidates to discover and eliminate (with occasional interventions by me) the reasons for Eberhard's tinnitus, which had suddenly begun a year earlier. The tinnitus was constantly present, in the left ear much worse than in the right one. He had already had an ear infection as a child. Let us begin again for the sake of simplicity with his life as a perpetrator.

Eberhard recognizes himself as Heinrich, the master of a German castle (Burg Grueneck) in the year 1180. He is fifty-one years old, but he has had no children with his wife, Katharina. There is war, as another castle-lord wants to take possession of his land. Heinrich's soldiers have taken numerous prisoners. They are now being tortured to gain confessions. They are tied up stretched to the wall or unpleasant liquids are poured with a funnel into their mouths. Heinrich enjoys these tortures and is watching this spectacle with satisfaction. At his own pleasure he also takes part in the torturing. He takes a bow and arrow, for instance, and shoots a tied man in his left ear to see how deep the arrow will go. The prisoner cries in anguish but dies very soon soon from the wound.

The callous Heinrich gives up his body at the age of seventy-four (*one could add that he then entered upon the journey to retribution that was to last till the 20th century*). His list of sins is outrageous. (*I would never want to load such a burden of karma upon myself. But perhaps I was also at some time no better – we all (at least most of us) seem to have been great sinners at some time or other.*)

Four of the karmic resolving earlier lives connected to his present tinnitus are investigated. In the first he is an Indian named Joni in the Brazilian jungle around 1342. He is a hunter armed with bow and arrow and despite his thirty-five years of age still unmarried. He loves being alone. But marriage seems to be rather unimportant in his tribe, as there they all sleep with each other anyway according to their mutual desires. On the day of his death, a cut-down tree falls on his neck, a branch jabbing into his left ear. He dies immediately, lying on his stomach. He also leaves the body right away and can describe from without the exact position of his body and of the tree.

In one of his next lives he is an Eskimo woman named Kiri, forty-four years old, with three children and an alcoholic husband. When the latter is drunk, he beats his wife and children. One time, again in this condition, he is about to start beating his children, but Kiri, their mother, tries to protect them. He throws her headfirst against the wall. Her head suddenly starts to buzz, and nausea overcomes her. She is dizzy, and pains in her neck start to spread into her head. Suddenly she cannot hear any longer, she sees the children crying and lies down on the floor. She can only see the mouth movements of her angry husband, but cannot understand what he is saying.

She is led to the day before her death. She is now sixty-two years old and still living with her husband, whom she hates. The children have left. Since the day of that accident she is deaf, so they only communicate by hand signs. The back of her neck still hurts, and she often has dizzy-spells and headaches.

In another life Eberhard is a forty-eight year-old man in Tunisia. It is 1834 and his name is Amir. He wears a turban and trades in camels. Amir falls off a camel and while falling is hit by its hoof on his left ear and jaw. His left jawbone is broken. Although he is treated, the jaw never heals. He dies at the age of sixty-seven from heart and breathing problems. Afterwards he sees how his body is laid in a box and covered with sand. It is interesting to note that some symptoms from which he now suffers were already present – his heart and respiratory problems. Whether these were karmic results of his life as Heinrich or results of other lives could not be investigated here.

And there was in another life as a victim a karmic cause for the problems with his left ear. In 1920 he was Jean, the owner of a Paris nightclub, who always kept 6-8 girls ready for his masculine customers. He was unmarried, but slept with his prostitutes. At the same time he was corrupt - and stingy, for which he was hated. When he was fifty-three, two men with pistols broke into his beautiful house, tied him up and hit him on the left cheek and ear with the butt of their guns to make him open the safe. After they had cleaned out the safe, one of them pointed his pistol at him, says, "You dirty pig!" and pulled the trigger. The bullet hit him directly below his left ear. He was dead immediately. The housekeeper, who came on account of the noise, was also shot. Jean, who was already outside of his body, saw the two bodies still bleeding from the head, heard the gangsters laugh and leave the house. His "never-again" sentence was formulated as follows: "I will never again cheat others. I will never again abuse women or degrade them sexually. I will never again misuse my power or be attached to wealth."

On the Mountain of Revelation Eberhard recognizes the causal effect of the law of karma and accepts it as just. After he has given the cup to all the others mistreated by Heinrich in his callousness and criminal brutality and asked for their forgiveness, he carries the Golden Cup to his soul as Heinrich, forgiving him too for what he has done.. Then he goes into his lives as a victim and forgives all those who caused him suffering. This all the easier for him now because he knows that he himself had chosen, for instance, the brutal husband of Kiri in order to attain karmic retribution through his mistreatment as the cause of her deafness.

It may often seem strange that women mistreated by their drunken husbands often remain with them instead of leaving. But they know subconsciously that they can attain through them at least a part of the karmic balancing that they have already "prescribed" for themselves in the beyond.

We can see therefore that through Regression Therapy completely new perspectives for psychology arise – and also of course for law. A few decades from now perhaps courts will delve into karmic backgrounds in order to reach more just decisions. Anyway, every strict decision in court, whether just or unjust, is the result of an earlier life as a perpetrator. Thus no court can make a wrong decision. But the judge and jury can burden themselves with karma if they make a decision conflicting with their own consciences. For as we have already seen long ago: everything that we do to others comes back to us in the form of karmic reactions.

Now Eberhard realizes, too, that the two murderers of Jean killed him for karmic reasons, so he can actually be grateful for them for helping balance his karma. Of course, that does not free them from the karmic reactions they will also meet some time. And, as we have seen, karmic balancing of his misdeeds in the life as a perpetrator in Middle Age Germany spread itself over the different parts of the world (South America, North America, Africa and Europe), only to return in the present life to Germany. The circle has been closed. We can also recognize in that a certain higher plan.

18. Every strike causes a karmic reaction (Neuralgia of the trigeminus)

Vera is a forty-five year-old civil servant in the finance ministry who suffers from acute case of trigeminus neuralgia, apparently incurable by neural therapy, acupuncture or homeopathy. To keep her life somehow on track she has psychiatric drugs prescribed regularly. The pain spreads over the right side of her face from above the eye down to the corner of her mouth. Sometimes the pain comes in surges, but at intervals of every 14 days or less, lasting then one to four days. During this time she takes painkillers. The pain is often accompanied by nausea, and in the acute phase she is unable to work. Then she has to recline most of the time. Being very undemanding, she only requires someone to be with her when she is in the acute phase. Usually it is possible for her husband, her son or a girl friend to accompany her at that time, otherwise she is constantly in tears.

But this neuralgia is only the main problem; she also is plagued by fear of the future, feelings of inferiority, fear of crowds, fear of loss, fear even of herself. Then there is obsessive perfectionism, the compulsive need to do everything at once, along with a helper syndrome – all symptoms of her dissatisfaction. She admits being sometimes arrogant and aggressive. And after the Regression Therapy session she admits having a violent hate of her stepfather, who often abused her sexually when she was a teenager. This was also tolerated by her mother.

In her life as a perpetrator Vera experiences herself as a thief in Paris in the year 1472, who is now sitting out his sentence in a dark prison, having been convicted of horse-stealing. Every day he is whipped. He has a violent hate for all wealthy people, so he sees it as his right to steal from them whenever he has a chance. After forty days he is released.

Later he becomes a pimp, living with the twenty-five year-old prostitute on whose proceeds he lives. He beats her when she does something he does not like, when she seems too lazy or too stupid to satisfy her customers or to take enough money from them. Generally he slaps her on the right cheek. When he again turns to stealing, he is caught by the gendarmes and shot in the back when he breaks away from their grip. The angry passers-by kick the dying man in the face and scream, "Bastard!"

Here the soul receives some of its karmic balancing in the same life: The pimp slaps his prostitute on the right cheek, and the crowd kicks him in the face as he is dying. But this is only a small part of the suffering the soul would still have to face. In fact it would be three hundred years until this soul was balanced, in the meantime having to experience a similar fate to that of the prostitute in his life as a perpetrator. Surely there are other things from that life that the soul will have made up for in the meantime. As we have already shown here in many cases, karmic balancing can take a long waiting time, but it will come in the long run. Even a slap on the cheek must be made up for in some way.

In 1791 this soul lives in Germany as a young woman named Sabine. She lives with her mother, a well-known town prostitute. Although the mother calls her daughter "ugly", she has forced her to sleep with men. At twenty years of age she goes to the well to get water, when she is spit upon by other women. Then children come, shouting, "Witch! Witch!" Finally, the women hold her fast, while one hits her face on the right wide with a stick until it is covered with blood.

Sabine goes the same day to the river with the intention of drowning herself. She feels herself to be guilty, inferior and sinful. Her face hurts; she looks awful. But she is afraid to end her life. Something keeps her from taking this last step. So she decides to leave town and go to Limburg, where she gets a job as a waitress. Later she marries – a happy but childless marriage.

After death, at seventy-three, her dead husband meets her, hugging her and leading her into the light. From her Higher Self she learns that her mother then is also her present mother, who allows her husband to sleep with Sabine to keep him from leaving her or turning to other women.

All the slaps that Sabine in her earlier life as a pimp gave to his prostitute were given back in the form of her being hit with a stick until bloody, perhaps even down to the exact same number of hits. And because the pimp had forced the girl to become a prostitute, he had to be reborn as Sabine in order to experience the same fate. But this obviously was not sufficient, so that Vera had to experience abuse from her stepfather, so as to – hopefully – finally erase the earlier misdeeds.

Her neuralgia comes from the connection between her life as a perpetrator and her lives as a victim, the latter still carrying over into the present life. This karma cannot be completely eliminated yet, for she learns from her Higher Self that she first will have to conquer her arrogance toward others. But a considerable improvement can now occur.

On the Mountain of Revelation some other connections are made clear to her: the origin of her fear of crowds was the ugly scene at the well, where the women held her and beat her in the face. This fear is also directly connected to the trigeminus neuralgia. I had supposed that the girl beaten by the pimp in the earlier life could be her present stepfather. But he was a woman in another life, who was badly treated by Vera when she was a man.

Because I can only offer the reader in this book a small selection of examples from Regression Therapy, I will have to leave out many other examples from my files referring to the various parts of the head. I only want to give the reader an impression of how previous misdeeds out of callousness can be represented in the present life as karmic symptoms and how they can be balanced out by Regression Therapy. But now I will give an example of karmic suffering in the neck area.

19. When karma strangles one within the same lifetime (Chronic problems of the neck and throat)

Gabriele was a ballet-dancer and is now head of training in a German ballet theater. She often had the feeling of being out of breath or even being strangled. Besides this, she often had throat aches. She had already visited me a year before, when we took care of her migraine and her teeth problems and discovered among other things three lives as a perpetrator. It had seemed to her to be a complete success, as her migraines as well as all her bothersome teeth problems had disappeared. Now she wanted also to rid herself of her neck problems and – if possible – also her personal love problems. She was namely good looking and single but somehow not able to develop a close relationship to a man. One of her greatest desires was to have a harmonious relationship.

In her life as a perpetrator she was a coarse man named Frank, thirty years old. In 1491 he traveled from place to place in Germany and was single, a fact that can partly be attributed to his addiction to sex. But he was an unpleasant fellow who seemed to know no limits. He had already raped several women and gotten away with it. But this time he took a prostitute to his hotel room, where they got into an argument. Frank then choked the woman and finally cut her throat. Fleeing again, this time he was caught and hanged.

In her life as a victim Gabriele is a twenty-five year old nun named Sophie. She lives in a French monastery in the year 1756. She comes from a very wealthy, aristocratic home, where she felt herself unloved both by her mother and by her father. Her mother, by whom she felt rejected, seemed completely foreign to her. Her father was seldom at home.

At seventeen she was sent to a boarding school, but she decided rather to enter a monastery. One day men came and demanded that Sophie come with them, as she had entered the monastery illegally, i.e. without the consent of her father. The latter had sent the messengers after procuring a consenting letter from the bishop.

The man who takes her from the monastery has been chosen as her husband by her father. He seems horribly ugly to her, is fifteen years older and also very wealthy. His name is Henry. After the marriage ceremony, when she has to share a bed with Henry, she notices that he smells of alcohol. She refuses him. He hits her and starts to strangle her (!). Afraid of him, from then on she lets him have his way. But still he seems to enjoy making her suffer physically. Luckily Henry is often away on business. She bears him two children.

Now fifty years of age, she is lying on her deathbed. I ask her to look back on her life and to tell me what she would do differently or never do again. She answers, "I will never again be silent. I have never defended myself. I will never again do something against my will. I will never again have a relationship with a man. I want to be alone." These last thoughts or feelings, whether expressed or silently thought, are the actual program for future experience. Therefore one should die free of such thoughts, for whatever has remained unsolved in life finds its sequel in following lives on earth.

Her last two sentences were taken into the life which now has taken place as Sophie in Germany. The program: "I want to be alone and I will not have a relationship with a man", has been completely fulfilled even in her today life. And without Regression Therapy it possibly would have been carried forward into other lives to come.

Her neck pains have to do with both of these lives. Again and again in Regression Therapy a problem or symptom is found to be coupled with a whole series of other symptoms and problems. The latter can also be cleared up through clearing up the former and passing the cup for them. Possibly in this case Gabriele will be able to live, too, in a satisfying relationship and even allow the man to touch her over-sensitive neck, because the neck is certainly free of pain and there should be no feeling of choking left.

Here we have another case in which the perpetrator (Frank) attains karmic balancing already in the same life by suffering the same or a similar fate – he suffers a death in which also his air is cut off. But with that the neck karma was not completely dissolved. As Sophie she was often choked. And one can easily imagine how terrible these experiences must have been, seeing that probably a certain neck phobia would have been carried over from the life as a perpetrator, even today still causing problems for Gabriele's neck, including frequent pains. Such pains are, as we will see, usually reminders of karmic causes that the soul has not yet cleared up. Their purpose is to remind us to finally take care of them.

In this case also a typical reaction behavior based on feelings of karmic guilt is demonstrated. After a life as a perpetrator a soul often chooses a life in renunciation, e.g. as a monk or nun, in the (subconscious) aim of doing penance, on the one hand, for guilt still burdening it from another life and, on the other, to attain a life position from which it is impossible to fall back into previous behavior patterns. So even lives as nuns can have a karmic background.

Before I had finished the final correction of the manuscript for this book, I was able to reach Gabriele by telephone. She told me that she had felt a greater inner stability since this Regression Therapy session and was living in a satisfying relationship. She had been even able – as a previous absolute teetotaler – to drink a beer now and again and – this was the most important result – had been free of neck pains and could even allow people to touch her neck which was before impossible for her to let it happen.

20. Dishonesty and karma (Backaches)

Rose is forty-two years old. She has borne two children, but even during her pregnancy her marriage was already a game of insincerity. Finally she got a divorce and has lived since then with a new partner in a harmonious relationship, attending together with him my training seminar in

Regression Therapy.

Shortly after the birth of her second child the back pains began, above all in the lower back. The doctor diagnosed a slipped disk and saw Rose's one-sided, carrying of her first child as the cause. With the birth of her second child the back pains often became intolerable, already beginning in the morning. Nursing the child was a real torture, but she refused to take any painkillers, against the advice of her doctor. And down to the present day these pains from the lower back all the way up to the back of the neck have not receded. As a demonstration example in my seminar, I led her back to the sources of her present back problems.

In her life as a perpetrator her name is Tonn, a thirty year-old man with unruly hair. He desires a woman a little older than himself, because she owns a lot of land. He is determined to marry her. But this woman, Sila, changes partners often, she cannot make up her mind which one to marry. Tonn hits her present lover in the back and strangles him from behind, then goes directly to her, demanding that she marry him and saying that he can protect her best. There was a festival below at the moment, that would be the best place to now proclaim their engagement. But Sila tells him that she does not like him and does not want to marry any man at present because she would like to be free for various relationships. But Tonn is bent on marrying her, although he does not love her either. He threatens her, finally beating her, so that she is permanently injured on her back and head. Tonn appears to have slipped into the house and can escape without being seen. Sila becomes mentally deranged from the attack, and Tonn becomes himself mentally ill at 75, dying three years later. Her Higher Self tells Rose that her soul as Tonn wanted to learn the lesson that one should never try to get anything by force. The soul of Sila is living in Rose's present life as a non-medical practitioner with whom she has a lot of contact.

In her first karmic balancing life as a victim she is a fifty-seven year-old man named Mustafa in Mongolia in the year 1632. He is the supervisor of ten women in a tannery and leather-working shop. Suddenly there is a great clamor when one of the women slips on the wet stones and falls off a cliff. He runs to look, but slips himself, too. Falling, he lands with his back on a stone and remains there unconscious. They carry him into a stone hut. Regaining consciousness, he feels strong pain in his head and above all in his back. Having broken a vertebra in his lower back, he has to use crutches for a half-year. Though often bedridden as a result of back pains, he lives a long life.

In the next karmic balancing life for her misdeeds as Tonn, Rose is a thirty-seven year old Catholic priest named Raphael in 1733 in Cologne. Secretly he has already had several affairs with women. At the moment he is standing at a tower window ready to jump to his death. He is in love with a woman but cannot marry her because of his vows as a priest. After many secret meetings with her, a priest never being allowed to be alone with a woman except when separated by a wall in the confessional, he finds himself in a great inner conflict between God, represented by the church, and his love for this woman. His heart belongs to the woman, but he is not allowed to love her, being bound to serve God all his life in chastity. Now he jumps, his back breaks on hitting the pavement and he dies immediately.

Most suicides still wander around this world after death, visiting those they have left behind to register their reactions. Everything seems to be controlled in a meaningful way from "above", in order to possibly reach an act of purification for those souls without an earthly body by helping them to regret their deed.

But Raphael seems to have been immediately taken into the beyond. He meets shining beings in a world of light. They apparently have been waiting for him. He believes he can read their minds. They lead him into a building with a white dome built under a waterfall. This falling water astounds him, flowing into the large pool in which he is now to sit. Here he experiences a purifying and relaxing effect through the power of the water.

Usually if we have experienced a brutal death, we are allowed to convalesce in a kind of sanatorium in the beyond, or, as here, to undergo a process of rejuvenation. Coming out of the water, he is asked to lie on the ground and stretch out his arms. He feels now how a beam of yellow light from above enters into his abdomen. Suddenly he sees his life as Rafael before him. He sees how, as a priest, he stands at the pulpit and tells lies, preaching chastity but not living it himself. He should have stood up to his inner self and left the Church, even if he had been threatened with death. He is confronted all at once very clearly with the hypocrisy of the Church, recognizing that he was himself entangled in it, making himself guilty, too. But it is also revealed to him from within that these lies are important as an experience. Because only through the lies – and their destructive power against love – can one become aware of the possibility of attaining the truth, even if only after death.

And these statements remind us of those above (*cf. hay fever, Case 2*) in which it was said that we must first become perpetrators in order to recognize our own loveless callousness and in the karmic balancing events that we ourselves have to endure as victims, finally attaining through them the experience of love. And in the same way it is possible that we have to first be led into experiences where we lie ourselves, then in karmic processes have to experience the same or similar lies in the same or following lives, until we have learned to stand up for our own inner truth, never again wavering from it and never lying again. To sum up: First you must experience, then balance out, then understand. Finally you your thinking, speaking and acting will be led by love and truth.

Rose's back problems were composed of two karmic components: Firstly, they were a result of her life as a perpetrator as Tonn, which required two lives as a victim – one as Mustafa and one as Rafael – through back ailments as karmic balancing factors. In the life as Rafael a new learning topic turned up under the theme "truth". In this way the back became a carrier for this theme. It combined itself with the theme, so much so that even in the present life they are still interwoven.

For, as Rose later confessed, she lived in and after her second pregnancy in a jungle of falsehoods with her husband. This was the basis for the worsening backaches. And later she also confessed that she had already lived as a young girl in a conflict between uprightness and dishonesty, having grown up in a monastery boarding school. She said that there she had to lie "as much as she possibly could", as she expressed it. These lies began already in the confessional. Bodily feelings of sense enjoyment were frowned upon and ignored. They were not even supposed to exist, and it was forbidden to speak about them. One was trained to lie, in complete contrast to the declared aim: to give school training to "pure and pious young virgins" and to prepare them for life. So she had also in present life been confronted at an early age with the theme "truthfulness".

We human beings are led into situations in which we are tested as to how far we can stand up for our inner truth and how far we have actually learned the lessons experienced in our karmic balancing events. So it is perhaps necessary – in case we have not learnt our lesson – again and again to be put in such a situation of being induced to lie, then in corresponding situations in which we suffer from the lies of others, and finally to undergo tests of our honesty.

As soon as we can live without lies and stand up for our inner truth, we will need no more tests on this point. But we may need tests on other things. Karma is the vehicle leading us to become upright and loving persons. Karma has no value of its own, but is a means to an end – an end well arranged from high above.

From her Higher Self Rose also learned that the woman she had loved as Raphael was her present partner. She could not yet be completely freed from her backaches, as she still had to work on these new revelations. But when she had finished this work, her backaches would totally disappear. Rose knew what was meant by that: still unfinished matters concerning her divorced husband. Afterwards, in fact, the more she consciously worked on herself, the more the backaches disappeared. And when she called again a year later, her backaches had totally disappeared.

Although in very many cases of Regression Therapy a complete or partial success results immediately, there are also cases in which according to the statements of the Higher Self the client will have to work further on him/herself or on the problem. In these cases complete success then usually takes place in its due time.

21. When karmic bullets hit their target (Heart cramps)

Orthodox medicine still tends to take a reserved or negative stance toward Regression Therapy. But that will certainly change soon, for the great numbers of successful treatments of this therapy method will not be possible to ignore much longer. Already a number of medical doctors have had me train them to become a regression therapist. In the following case we have to do with a medical doctor who is also a psychiatrist and psychotherapist.

Because a number of traditional methods proved themselves unable to offer him lasting relief from his heart problem and neurodermatitis, he decided to try Regression Therapy. Neurodermatitis has been present on his cheeks and forehead for the past ten years. Kenneth, as I want to call him, believes that psychic problems could play a part, as he has a fear of failure as well as a fear of closeness. He also finds it difficult to accept help from others. He had an Oedipal conflict with his father and loved his mother. But she was a borderline-case, being full of ambivalences and often threatening to commit suicide. In addition he had an inexplicable hate of the color purple. So he wanted to finally discover the reasons behind all these symptoms. Thus we left it up to his Higher Self to choose what to reveal to him in the Regression Therapy session.

In the first life revealed to him, Kenneth was a French Franciscan monk named Samuel in the year 1512. He describes his life: He goes to bed at ten o'clock and is already at morning prayers by daybreak. He had entered the monastery at the age of twenty-eight because he found no love in the world and wanted then to find love of God. Now he is thirty and is driving to a farm where the ox-cart full of barrels he has with him are to be filled with grain. He is familiar with the farm from the previous years, but when he arrives, he finds there everything destroyed and most of the buildings burnt down. The chickens, pigs, cat and dog come to him hungry. Samuel has to cry at this sight. Then he discovers upon walking through the remains a three year-old boy, his face full of smut. Suddenly also an old man appears, who has survived the inferno. He tells Samuel that a band of men, some of them dressed in animal skins, had come and killed all the men present, whom he has already buried. The women were then abducted.

The old man allows Samuel to take the boy, his grandson, and care for him. Even later the feeling of personal guilt for what happened to the farm never leaves him. (I was never able to find out the reason for this guilt.)

The boy grows up among the monks but leaves the monastery at the age of twenty-eight, sailing to North Africa. Samuel himself catches leprosy in Spain at seventy. The sores spread over his face. The country itself was at war with the Arabs and everywhere there was destruction. An Arabian doctor gave him water alleged to be a cure, which Samuel wiped over his sores. And in fact they disappeared after a while, leaving scars. At eighty-two he died in his sleep.

After death Samuel finds himself all at once on a meadow full of flowers. Here he meets a small girl. Suddenly he meets the old man again whose grandson he has taken in. Samuel belongs to a group of twelve to thirteen souls who seem as familiar as members of his own family and some of whom he knows or thinks he knows from his past lives. At the Gate of Clouds he hears from his Higher Self that he had to experience leprosy for karmic reasons, which are also the cause for his present neurodermatitis. And now we asked his Higher Self to show us the cause for Kenneth's heart problem.

He experiences himself immediately as Francois, a nineteen year-old French law-student from Lyon. He is studying in Nantes, but in 1914, at the outbreak of war, he immediately joins the military. During an attack on the enemy front he is shot in the heart. Suddenly he is floating over his body, sees many dead bodies beneath and also their spirit bodies floating around him. In a cloud they are all taken to a country house, where each of them gets his own room to rest in. As Francois awakens, an angel-like woman calling herself Martinique stands next to his bed. She answers his question as to where he is by telling him that he is in heaven. They seem to have understood each other so well that Martinique wanted to become his wife in his next life (*i.e. the present one*).

In the next life we investigate Kenneth sees himself as a Syrian Jew named Aron in the year 652 (*possibly according to the Arabian time-system*). He is a shoemaker, married, with a daughter. The church in the city has just been burned down by unknown persons. The Jews are given the blame. A pogrom begins in which many Jews lose their lives. Furthermore it was ordered that Jews no longer may carry out trades, send their children to school or lock their doors. Thus anyone may enter their houses at any time to attack their women or steal something. Aron's wife is also raped during this pogrom.

A cardinal in purple robes enters the city. Aron, who now lives from begging – he has already lost everything – takes heart, pushes through the crowd and falls at the feet of the cardinal, raising his arms pleadingly and saying that the Jews are being wrongly persecuted. But the cardinal pushes him aside contemptuously with his staff. Aron cries out, "We Jews are also humans, just as you are a human." But then soldiers come to kick him, so he quickly escapes into the crowd. Later he is able to escape to Crete with his family, where he can take up shoemaking again. He dies at seventy-eight.

According to his Higher Self, his life as Aron was necessary for karmic reasons. And his distaste for purple comes from the robe of the cardinal who pushed him aside. But also his fear of loss – including the feeling of being rejected – is a karmic remnant of this life as Aron.

Now I requested Kenneth to ask his Higher Self to lead him into the life that had been the cause for his heart-wound as Francois. And the Higher Self sent him through another Gate of Clouds.

He realizes himself as a thirty-nine year-old French Lieutenant of Italian descent named Jean. He was at that time – the year 1815 – in Savoy, where 250 soldiers were under his command. Another officer had offended him, and Jean challenged him to a duel. The fencing duel takes place on an empty street. After the other officers form a circle, the opponents take their caps off and begin to duel. Jean's opponent is injured and falls. Jean takes advantage of the opportunity – although his opponent is already disabled – and stabs him deep in the heart. On the one hand he is proud of his victory, on the other frightened. Accompanied by his friends, he goes to a tavern. He is afraid of perhaps being called to account and punished for the duel by higher officers, but nothing happens.

So this was the reason for his karmic balancing life as a victim as Francois in the First World War, and the place where the bullet hit was the exact same place where Jean had jabbed his opponent wtth the pointed weapon. We should actually be astounded that karmic balancing often occurs on the body at the same place as the original wound, arousing the question: "Who guides the weapons so that the same places are hit?" In other words there must be higher arrangers, otherwise how should the bullet know that it is supposed to bring about karmic balancing by hitting Francois' heart?

Is everything predetermined? We have also already seen that one chooses one's coming fate oneself. But even so there must be such super-intelligent beings to set up or carry out the processes that we have planned ourselves before entering a new earth life. Are then all bullets seeking their victims on the battlefield predetermined? If this is so, there must be thousands of invisible entities carrying out karmic processes on each and every battlefield to lead every bullet to the pre-established target – without perhaps hitting someone else by accident. And on the other hand those who are not hit by bullets are protected from such a fate – because they have so chosen in the beyond. A great number of such questions press themselves upon us. We will have an opportunity later to go into some of them more deeply.

Kenneth realized these karmic connections very clearly on the Mountain of Revelation. After this very successful Regression Therapy session, his heart problems may now have disappeared, for their cause has been revealed. He forgave the German who shot him in the heart, just as he asked his dueling-opponent for forgiveness – his present brother-in-law – offering him the Golden Cup of forgiveness and love.

A year later I called Kenneth to ask him about his condition. I was very glad to hear that his heart was in relatively good shape – by which he was astounded – but not completely well. Not only was his heart in better shape, but also his high blood pressure had improved, allowing him to reduce the amount of medicine he used. In general he was experiencing, as he said, "a friendlier relationship with his heart." Respecting his neurodermatitis, the causes of which we had only discovered a few (though important ones), there had also been a substantial improvement. The earlier drastic symptoms had not reappeared. "In any case," as he said, he had experienced "an improvement". I am convinced that after one or two more Regression Therapy sessions he would be completely free of all his heart and skin problems.

Traversing the body from top to bottom in search of karmic sources of somatic illnesses, we now come to the abdomen.

22. How karma "hounds" its victims (Stomachaches)

Elisabeth is thirty-six years of age, divorced and mother of one son. She is a nurse, but has now begun training to become a healing practitioner. (Usually non-medical practitioners come to me after finishing their exams.) Admitting to having a helper syndrome, she can hardly refuse anyone's wishes.

Elisabeth has suffered since she was fourteen from chronic stomachaches that she claims have nothing to do with her menstruation. Previously only occurring every few days, for the past few years they have been constant. She has undergone no operations yet, but there have been many medical examinations to determine their cause and nature. Because the pains wander throughout the whole abdominal region from one place to the next, they are variously diagnosed as kidney cysts, weakness of the stomach closure-muscle, growths on the gall bladder or twisting of the intestine.

Besides these somatic symptoms, Elisabeth suffers without reason from the belief that she is not pretty enough and therefore unable to find someone to love or desire her. She is afraid of being made fun of and afraid of being alone.

I then demonstrate to the participants of the seminar how to find the causes of such abdominal pains, possibly attaining an immediate cure.

She experienced herself in 1817 as a nineteen year-old Dutch girl named Annemarie, the daughter of a politically influential man. It is dark already and she is on the way to visit her boyfriend Matthias. Suddenly she is grabbed from behind, thrown on the ground. Two men hit her in the stomach with iron bars, then disappear into the darkness. She is later found covered with blood and carried home, where she dies in the arms of her father, for whom she was the most beloved possession. After death she finds herself on a flowery meadow. At the Gate of Clouds Elisabeth learns from her Higher Self that political enemies wanted to take revenge on her father by having hired assassins take his most precious possession. When her Higher Self was asked if there was any other causal life for her abdominal pains, the answer was no. So we asked it to lead us to a life in which the cause for her having to die as Annemarie could be found.

Elisabeth is a thirty-two year-old Hungarian man named Joerg. (*He called himself "Joerg". Perhaps his real name was "Gyorgy", which would be equivalent to the German name "Joerg". As we have mentioned above, often the equivalent native name is given for the foreign one: e.g. Robert for Roberto, Maria for Mary and Hans for Jean. But of course also many Germans lived at that time in Hungary and they had also German names.*) His former friend Markus has stolen his girlfriend Julia from him. When he sees them walking together, they turn around and laugh at him. Because Markus is a nice-looking young man, Joerg believes that his attractiveness was responsible for his conquest. Jealous, he decides to kill his rival. He waits for him in the dark and stabs him several times in the stomach. Running away, Joerg washes the blood from his hands, face and clothes at a well and then goes to his friend Harald's house. The prime suspect, Joerg is arrested and interrogated. But Harald claims that Joerg had been playing cards with him all night. Meeting Joerg later on the street, Julia accuses him, but Joerg answers cynically, "Now I have the last laugh."

Remaining single, he suffers from loneliness and feels himself too ugly to try to court women. When asked before his death if he regrets anything, he says, "No." Nevertheless he admits that he is afraid of eventually being punished by a higher authority. (*Here are two of the reasons for Elisabeth's present fear of being alone and for her ugliness complex. The latter problem at least is without foundation, for many women would be glad to have only a portion of her beauty and attractiveness.*)

After his death at the age of seventy, he sees his body lying on a bench – apparently he has died of heart failure.

When asked for his I-will-never-again sentence, he replies, "I will never again be made fun of. I never want to be ugly again." (*Here he still has no regrets, otherwise he would have said, "I will never again be jealous. I will never again kill anyone" etc. - Here we also recognize where Elisabeth's fear of ridicule originates.*)

When he is asked to find the next important event after his death, he suddenly meets Markus, who greets him with an open handshake, saying, "Joerg, I am not angry with you."

Perhaps some explanation is necessary here. Markus has already been in the beyond for forty years. Of course he will have learned already that his own death at the hand of Joerg had a karmic justification, for no one can kill anyone else who does not "deserve" death on karmic grounds and has even chosen this fate. Markus is even thankful for this karmic balancing event. And at the same time he feels empathy for Joerg, who will also have to let himself be murdered. If someone remains in the beyond for a long period of time like Markus, he does it in order to learn a great deal about the spiritual laws. Perhaps he wanted to remain there until Joerg came. But of course he also could have incarnated one or two times in the meantime. At any rate he uses his form as Markus so that he can be recognized by Joerg.

Joerg is suddenly overcome with feelings of guilt. (*And they were to remain with him until his present life.*) It is incomprehensible for him that his victim is not angry at him. Instead Markus puts his arm around Joerg's shoulder and says, "Come, I want to show you something." He leads Joerg to a dried-up meadow, where he leaves him. (*Murderers and other evil characters are usually greeted by someone and led to a dark area or – as in this case – to a deserted, dreary area, which mirrors at the same time their own dark or impure character. They then remain there until they recognize and regret their mistakes. As soon as that has happened – the length of time required is irrelevant – one of the wise persons comes and leads them out of this hell that such persons have created for themselves by their misdeeds and callous attitude on earth.*)

After he has recognized his mistakes and his loveless attitude on earth, Joerg is met by a person dressed in white and carrying a staff with a ball on top. He tells him, "You can come with me to a more beautiful country, as soon as you have learned to regret." And Joerg expresses again his deeply felt regret, even kneeing down and praying for forgiveness for all the evil deeds done in his life on earth. The figure in white leads him now into a room filled with a fog-like substance and covered with a glass dome. Here he is given shining new clothes that he puts on after taking off his dirty old rags. Suddenly his body begins to shine brightly. And his companion, seeing how skeptical and bewildered the still guilt-conscious Joerg appears, says, "You shouldn't be so dissatisfied with yourself." Joerg feels great relief within and hears a voice saying to him, "Do good in another life!" Joerg is suddenly overwhelmed with joy for being allowed to make up for his misdeed by doing something positive. (*This is the basis for his helper syndrome!*)

This may sound like a fairy-tale to the reader who has never had contact with what I am reporting here, but it is absolute fact! Even Elisabeth had, as she confessed to me later, never heard or read anything like it. But when we are confronted again and again with such descriptions in Regression Therapy – even from those who have never read or heard descriptions of the beyond – these transcriptions of trance experiences make a deep impression on us, gradually making us ask ourselves if there might be some truth in these statements. The truth is hidden behind many veils, and we humans know so little of it. But while advancing further in the future we will surely be able to lift one veil after the other, for this seems to be the destiny of mankind. And certainly Regression Therapy is in the process of raising one new veil, now already transparent, from the hidden surprises of creation.

Elisabeth now learns from her Higher Self that Julia is her present grandmother, Harald a girl friend and Markus missing in her present life. Furthermore, she is told that no other lives are needed to resolve her abdominal pains. She then places the contents mentioned in the following statement in her pinecone, saying, "I free myself of all feelings of guilt, from my fear of being alone. I free myself of my abdominal pains, my fear of being ridiculed. I free myself of my fear of not being loved and not being beautiful enough."

Immediately after the session Elisabeth noticed to her own amazement that the abdomen pains, still greatly noticeable up to that point, had now disappeared. And when I spoke with her on the telephone a half-year later, she told me they had not returned, adding also that she had been completely satisfied with herself since the session and had no longer felt any hate of anyone, not even of her ex-husband, nor fear of being ridiculed. She felt sure of herself in standing up for her own opinions. She found herself suddenly attractive, saying, "Men are surrounding me like bees." Finally she said, "I am now simply happy!"

At the same seminar with Elisabeth there was another non-medical practitioner and ex-geologist who in the next demonstration session would also be freed from his ills.

23. When the skin "cries" for karma balancing (Psoriasis)

Tony is forty-seven and divorced. He and his former wife have three children. In the previous year he was freed of claustrophobia in a Regression Therapy session. In one life as a victim he was a girl locked up in a room. When the house then caught on fire, she could not escape. He suffers from psoriasis, a kind of dandruff. The skin begins to turn red, and then scales begin to appear and then dry out. Finally, because of unbearable itching, one begins to scratch, causing moisture. And then the process begins anew. Psoriasis spreads over different parts of the body. Most unbearable is, perhaps, the affliction on the scalp, where there is a lot of scaling and dandruff. But this skin disease spreads out also on other parts of the head, on the back as well as the genital and anal area.

For Tony this all began at the age of twenty, at the same time as a boil began to develop in the anal area. He was reluctant to see a doctor until the age of 25, when the growth had reached the size of a pigeon egg and he had no other choice. The doctor gave him medicine, which did stop the growth of the boil but also caused the psoriasis to develop. The itching was worst whenever his wife or children came too close. (*This type of symptom is an alarm signal to a regression therapist to investigate whether one or more of these family members have a karmic connection with the actual cause in an earlier life as a victim or perpetrator.*)

First we went into his present life to see if there were things that could be seen in connection with his skin disease: At the age of three Tony burnt his hand on a candle. Going back to the age of one, we find him screaming in his baby-bed. His father, whose dentist's office is directly beneath this room, hears the cries and hurries upstairs, where he finds the baby-sitter missing. So he is forced to quickly change Tony's diapers himself. In his hurry he fails to put enough powder on the sore places before he hurries back to his office, scolding the reappearing baby-sitter on the way out.

Now I ask his Higher Self, if there is anything important for his skin problem in the prenatal period. He then experiences the moment when his mother learns that she is pregnant. She criticizes her husband for being at fault, saying, "It's just because you want to sleep with me all the time." The embryo Tony knows now that he is unwanted and would prefer, as he says, "to return to where he came from". Whenever his mother eats fruit, his skin burns.

So Tony can already suffer as a fetus. As we will see more clearly later, these are in fact (pre-selected) painful after-effects of karmic reactions in his life as a victim. Regression therapists have discovered this new fact: one can re-experience his life while in the womb as well as the whole process of one's birth through Regression Therapy.

At this point I led Tony to the moment of his birth. He experiences how his body is raised by a hand in a rubber glove and given a slap on the back. His body is completely blood-covered; his skin is sore all over and has to be treated immediately. His Higher Self tells us before the Gate of Clouds that these symptoms were due to the placenta water being full of acid from the berries eaten by his mother. (*It should therefore be tested – by kinesiological or other methods – what foodstuffs can be taken during pregnancy without causing suffering to the embryo or fetus. Or must the fetus suffer these pains on karmic grounds?!*)

And now we were again before the Gate of Clouds

asking his Higher Self to lead us to the real reason for his psoriasis: Tony experiences himself as a French field general named Frédéric Coulombat under Louis XIV. It is now 1706, and he is engaged in a battle with the English. Frédéric is married and has children, but, as we later learn, he does not love his family, preferring solitude instead. Against his will he has been made a general in the French army, and at the moment his troops are on the defensive, trying to reach a harbor (*perhaps in Belgium*) from which they are cut off.

Now Frédéric's horse is hit by a cannonball, causing both horse and rider to fall to the ground, where Frédéric is hit by burning tar from a projectile. His clothes, his hair, everything begins to burn. He is lying with one leg under the horse and cannot get free. The burning tar scorches his skin. Feeling terrible pain, he soon finds himself outside the body, from where he looks over the battlefield and sees his own body, charred and black. It seems to him that it was his own fault to put his soldiers needlessly in such a dangerous position, and he says, "I will never again take the responsibility for so many people." From his Higher Self he learns that his wife and child of that time, whom he was already afraid to be near, are his present mother and wife respectively.

In his next life Tony experiences himself as a nineteen year-old single woman named Sophia. She lives with an old man in a hut on a volcanic island in the South Seas. Feeling lonely, she occupies herself with making baskets out of rushes, while the old man keeps busy by making arrows.

On the day in question the cause for Tony's skin problems becomes apparent: Suddenly the ground shakes. The volcano is erupting. Day becomes night as the volcanic ashes darken the whole sky. The island-dwellers can hardly breathe, while loose rocks are flying through the air. They all assemble on the beach, and some consider going out with boots. But here they have at least some protection from the trees, whereas there they would surely fall prey to the flying stones. Then the lava comes pouring at great speed down the mountain. Many of them now seek safety in the water from the glowing red lava, but there is no escape. Her feet caught by the fiery, paste-like liquid, Sophia falls into the burning lava and is charred.

She learns from her Higher Self that the old man she lived with then is her present father. Tony has no contact today to the other dwellers of the island, but they may be all people who suffer from skin problems. *Does that mean that other people who suffer from psoriasis also have some karmic debt to pay from a former life and also have suffered burns? We will have to perform Regression Therapy with quite a number of people with such a skin problem to be able to make a final judgment. As we see, there is still a lot to be done in the discovery of karmic connections governing our lives.*

Led again before the Gate of Clouds, we asked his Higher Self to take Tony now into that life that was the real cause for the three lives where he was burnt to death. (*One had already turned up in the Regression Therapy of the year before*). There he perceived himself as an Irish fisherman named Hengar about the year 1500, who, in rage or revenge, set fire secretly to fields and even houses. In one of these arson attacks he was careless, even allowing his own hut to be caught by the flames, thus destroying also his wife and both children. Probably for this reason it was that he was never suspected.

On the Mountain of Revelation Tony recognizes the

connections very clearly and sees that for karmic reasons he had to die three times in the flames and suffer in his present life from a burning skin, too. His Higher Self points out to him that his wife and oldest son in his present life were also the wife and one of the sons he burnt to death then. Now he understands why he has to scratch himself whenever they come near him. (His wife is present when he visits his children two or three times a week at her house.)

As we will see later, there is a certain distinctive frequency "broadcast" subconsciously by everyone. It remains constant through one's life, allowing different souls to subconsciously recognize each other when they meet again. Both these family members broadcast, too, that frequency from the earlier life, so as soon as Tony comes close, his skin itches and he has to scratch himself. Upon meeting persons we are often subconsciously reminded of occurrences in earlier lives, and, if at those times they or we suffered injury to a certain part of the body, we may have an unpleasant feeling there. If we ourselves were responsible for those injuries, we may also be disturbed by the unavoidable feeling of guilt like the one that had accompanied Tony since the time he met his wife and married her.

But there was something else revealed to Tony by his Higher Self. If he had not had this illness in this life, he would never have taken up the path of spirituality. While mentally occupied with his illness he realized that there must be an inner cause for it and that he should not look without, but rather within, to cure it. Therefore he gave up his geological studies (*i.e. "looking without"*), became a Reiki-master and finally a non-medical practitioner in order to go the way of inner knowledge.

This sign given by his Higher Self is very significant. Are karmic illnesses meant to be positive, to help us move in the direction of finding our own center, i.e. our own soul? It must be clear that illnesses often bring about a change in people, changing their chronic high spirits, vanity and pride into humility. Thus karma brings about not only the realization of unsolved problems from earlier times – with the emphatic demand to understand and clear oneself of them. It also opens – by means of a painful symptom forcing an intensive confrontation – the gateway to one's own soul. I could imagine that the concept of karma holds the key not only to new inspiration for medical science as a whole, but also to a revolution within psychology, in particular. Hopefully the field of psychology will soon occupy itself as intensively with Regression Therapy as it now does even today with Freudian theory. These new discoveries of Regression Therapy force us to take a new "quantum-leap" in medicine and psychology.

Tony attended one of my supervision seminars a half-year later, where he told me that his psoriasis had improved by about 98%. His skin problems used to bother him especially in winter because of the dry air in heated rooms. But in that winter he had hardly felt an itch.

24. When karma is attached to a trigger (Hemorrhoids)

Karl is a globetrotter. He is sixty years of age, unmarried and a former teacher of history and German. Now he gives lectures and seminars on esoteric subjects. He has learned to apply reincarnation therapy on himself to rid himself of karmic burdens. Here is his report:

When I was a student in school and visited my

grandmother in the school vacations, I would always get hemorrhoids. She had grown up as a farmer's daughter and there was always lots of milk, curds and cheese to eat. But as soon as I returned to my boarding school the pains in my anus would stop.

During my college days I would cook myself a milk soup every morning and eat various other milk products during the day. The result was that I again got hemorrhoids which constipated me for days at a time. It was sometimes very difficult to pass stool, sometimes only with loss of blood and great painfulness, even once loss of consciousness.

Of course I went to the doctor's and got laxatives and other medicine to relieve my condition. But I was never asked about my eating habits. While walking I would sometimes get such a bad cramp in my anus that I could not walk any longer and had to wait five to ten minutes before being able to continue without extreme pain.

After my university studies, I traveled around the world as a hitchhiker, but never had hemorrhoids, because in the warmer countries milk products are hardly eaten. But then I arrived in the "land of milk and honey": in New Zealand I drank a whole liter of milk every morning, ate cheese and curds, whereupon I immediately got hemorrhoids again They were so bad that I had to consult a physician, who sent me to a surgeon. The surgeon ordered an immediate operation. The success of the operation allowed me to travel on to other warmer countries of the world, where I had no further pains. But I still had not seen a connection between this problem and dairy products.

After many years abroad I returned to my native country, finding work in an antique bookstore run by a friend of mine from university days. Noticing a return of my hemorrhoids, I mentioned it to him. He replied that he had had the same experience for many years, until a doctor told him to stop taking any dairy products. Upon following his advice, I was immediately relieved of my hemorrhoid condition. Suddenly the connection was clear. After that I took milk products only in minimal amounts – some milk or cream in my coffee – and experienced no reoccurrence of the problem.

But when I learned to use Regression Therapy and applied it also to myself, I decided to discover the causes of my former hemorrhoids. For it was clear to me that if I did not clear this up in my present life, it would return to me in the next. I put myself into the alpha-state and asked my Higher Self to lead me to the source of my hemorrhoids.

Suddenly I saw myself as a farmer's son of about thirty years of age, sitting in a stable and milking a cow. It could have been in Germany in the 17th century. Suddenly there was a great noise outside, and three vagabonds in tattered uniforms pushed the gate open, grabbed me from my stool, knocking the milk-bucket over and wetting the pitchfork lying there with the spilled milk. Then they grabbed me roughly by the arms, threatening to harm me if I did not tell them immediately where my money and silver were hidden. Because of the war ridden times I lacked both and therefore declared that I had no hidden reserves. "Yes, you have buried it. We will now force you to show your hideaway," the ruffians said. Again and again I stated that I myself was poor and had hidden nothing. Then they pulled down my trousers, made me bend over, took the still wet pitchfork and shoved the handle up my anus. Screaming with pain, I fell over unconscious. When I returned to consciousness I was lying in a puddle of blood. The villains had however left the farm.

Now I had found the cause of my hemorrhoids. But I also wanted to know why I had to experience this fate. After again entering the alpha-state and asking my Higher Self to lead me to the original cause of my hemorrhoids, I saw myself suddenly as a Tibetan man named something like "Ando" – of about the same age as the young German farmer – dressed in a fur hat and open blue jacket. I was married and supported myself and my wife – we seemed to have no children – by raising cattle and sheep. I had engaged several five to eight year-old boys to watch after my animals on the mountainsides. I liked to stay with these boys and forced them to sexual activities. I put my penis in their anuses against their will, the pain causing them often to cry or scream.

Now I had found the original cause of the karmic reactions. They were a similar kind as those suffered in the life as a German farmer and were still evident as repercussions in my present life. What occurred to me later was that I could never even imagine carrying out sexual practices with a boy, or even to practice anal sexuality with a woman – some inner repulsion forbids me from it. At that time I probably initiated a subconscious program never again to carry out anal sex.

After I offered as the young farmer the Golden Cup of reconciliation to the three ruffians at the end of that Regression Therapy session, I discovered that I suddenly could again consume any amount of diary products without ever again suffering from hemorrhoids. That is really a miracle! Possibly I took so long to find someone to awaken me to the connection between milk and my hemorrhoids because I had also in my present life still karma to suffer, karma left over from the life as a young farmer. So this was Karl's report.

Karl was also able to free himself from hemorrhoids by discovering the causes and receiving and giving forgiveness with the Golden Cup. This kind of self-treatment is, however, only advisable for those who know the process of Regression Therapy intimately and have the necessary self-confidence and courage to face their lives as a victim and a perpetrator alone.

So Karl had no milk-allergy, as one would have supposed. The milk was just a sign that there was a still unbalanced karmic disharmony in his anus. If he had died in an earlier life on poisoned milk, he certainly would have had a milk-allergy in his present life. Because everything has a specific frequency, the emotional body of the farmer connected the frequency of the milk with the pain caused by the pitchfork. His soul, which later incarnated as Karl, had stored at exactly the same place the information that something had still to be balanced. When Karl drank milk the related place in the emotional body began to resonate. These vibrations then were passed on the physical body, causing the painful hemorrhoids.

As soon as the person is led in Regression Therapy to the place and time of the original trigger and the connected karmic events are balanced, the injured place in the emotional body recuperates. In this case the milk was not the cause for the hemorrhoids, but a karmic "reminder", a messenger transmitting information to a place still in need of karmic rebalancing. After Regression Therapy it no longer had a receiver for its frequency.

But of course there can be also other causes of hemorrhoids. Future medical research will have the task of discovering the (perhaps many different) karmic causes of hemorrhoids. And when the respective lives as a perpetrator are entered into, one will often find forced anal sexuality as a primary causal event in the development of hemorrhoids manifesting itself in a later, perhaps even in the present life.

Every case of suffering caused to others out of one's personal interest boomerangs later as suffering for oneself. And hemorrhoids are only one among thousands of different causes of karmic pain. Now if every detail seems to be subservient to a higher plan or one's own plan, we could now ask critically, "Did that milk have to be poured intentionally over the pitchfork in order to act later as the effective carrier or trigger of karmic balancing events? Was this already foreseen and pre-planned? And is, as the Roman philosopher Plotinus claimed, everything that happens on earth already pre-established? Philosophers attempting to understand the foundations of karmic events will have to muse over such questions.

But let us now turn to a case in which karma affected almost the whole body.

25. When the present life becomes a place of karmic balancing (Muscular dystrophy)

Willy is fifty years old, and the past thirty-four of these years he has had to sit in a wheel chair. The diagnosis was "muscular dystrophy", i.e. disappearance of muscle tissue. At the age of one and a half years of age this began with weakness of the leg muscles. Gradually this increased, so that Willy was able to walk less and less the older he became. At the age of sixteen he was only able to take a few short steps, and from then on he was only able to move in his wheel chair. But this development was not only limited to the legs but spread out over the whole body. Today Willy can hardly even move his arms.

Besides this ailment he has also been bothered since childhood by feelings of guilt caused by his mother's death of blood-loss from the caesarian operation through which he was born. Other symptoms accompanied his muscular dystrophy such as speech and bladder disorders as well as chronic bronchitis. He is also afraid of being left alone and helpless.

At the age of twenty he met his wife Irmgard. She was on a walk with her girlfriend – they were visiting her grandmother for the Christmas holiday – when she saw the portrait of a blonde young man in the show-window of a photo shop. Stopping as if held by an invisible hand, she gazed at the picture and told her companion, "I could fall in love at once with that man. I would marry him right away."

After sitting up till midnight on New Year's with her grandmother, she went with her girlfriend to a dance. It was full, and there seemed to be no place left for the two girls to sit. But a young man saw the two nice-looking nineteen year-old girls, showing them the way to a long table, where he asked the other men to make room for them. After the two had seated themselves, Irmgard stared into the face of the man next to her. It was Willy, whose face she had seen in the photo shop. Their conversation was lively, and she wondered why he did not ask her to dance. As she said later, she felt attracted to him as if pulled by invisible powers. Willy asked her again and again to visit him at home, which she found strange. It would be improper, she thought, for a girl to chase after a boy by visiting him at home. Not until the dance was nearing an end and they said goodbye to each other did the situation become clear: two of the young men picked Willy up and put him in a wheel chair. And she kept her promise to visit him. A year later they were married.

The reason for my going into this strangely evolving romance will become clear in the previous lives that were to be investigated. For, as the reader has probably already guessed, we have to do here with a karmic relationship initiated as if by an invisible hand.

Willy had been writing novels since he was twelve years old, and by the age of twenty he was already a celebrated science-fiction writer. The strange events leading up to his marriage to Irmgard began to make him wonder whether higher or former connections had not perhaps played a part. They both began to occupy themselves with esoteric knowledge, finally opening up an esoteric bookstore.

In the first life opened to him by his Higher Self Willy is a physician named Tavion in ancient Greece in 783 B.C. He wears a white toga, is unmarried and about forty years of age and is in charge of a field hospital spread out in an olive grove near a temple. There are many patients there, most of them suffering from the plague. Tavion falls in love with a young woman also suffering from plague. But despite many months of feverish efforts to save her, she dies, leaving him depressed and immeasurably sad that he, as a doctor, was not able to save her. He leaves this hospital, draws back from all medical activity and dies soon afterwards from grief and despair.

After death he finds himself surrounded by light. The contours of entities are only vaguely recognizable. Suddenly he finds himself gazing into the face of his dead loved-one. He is floating with her in a kind of reception room. In this temple of light he can see through the walls, though they do not seem to be made of glass. He finds himself with his loved-one in a larger group of souls who all somehow seem to be acquainted with one another.

Arriving again at the Gate of Clouds, he learns from his Higher Self that that lover is Irmgard in his present life, who has dedicated herself to helping him in this life, so that she can reward him for his efforts to save her in his life as Tavion. But she has also another reason: she has to make up for suffering caused him in a different life by serving him in this life.

As we will also later see in other cases, souls are often reunited – whether on their own initiative or not - out of thankfulness or indebtedness in order to continue old karmic relationships in love or service. So-called "love at first sight" is usually a sign of love relationships from previous lives.

After being asked for the causes of Willy's dystrophy, his Higher Self leads him into a life as the head of a group of Russian soldiers in 1582. His name is Ankor and he is married to Nora, who bore him two children. They are now at war with another people, many of whom Ankor has already killed with his own sword. A day later at a great table on a nearby mountain the victory celebration is held, where alcohol flows in streams. Later at sixty he is a celebrated general, highly praised by his feudal lord, Prince Nikolaus, for having won many battles. After his death at seventy, he sees Nora and others standing around his body.

When asked about his "never-again" sentence, he answers promptly, "I will never again fight." This is a sentence spoken in Regression Therapy sessions by many persons who are today either pacifists, have weak bodies or are considered too soft and passive by their friends. For this program brings about a manifestation in reality and – as we see in this example – even on the body. Programming of this kind often takes effect for many lives, until other programs take over. For Willy they had the effect of making him helpless, the opposite of a physically active warrior. In front of the Gate of Clouds Willy learns that Nora is also his present wife, Irmgard. He had used his powers falsely in that life by destroying or maiming persons in battle. But there was also another life relevant to his present muscular dystrophy.

His Higher Self now leads him into this life. He sees himself as a muscular man of twenty named Butu, wearing a fur loincloth, who has already killed many warriors in battle with his club. When he is thirty-three, other warriors overrun his place. They hit him with their clubs all over his body, until he collapses and dies.

At the Gate of Clouds, back in his consciousness as Willy, he is told that the body is not so important. The main purpose is mental and spiritual development. If he had had a healthy body in this life, he would have missed another chance to develop himself spiritually. His illness had caused him to reflect on his life, benefiting him greatly. His wife had joined him out of love in this life in order to repay his earlier love for her with her own love.

Willy recognizes on the Mountain of Revelation the revealed karmic connections. He knows that his present life is karmic retribution for his previous callous killing of others. These discoveries will not make his muscles strong and healthy again all at once. Or perhaps I am wrong! We will see. In any case Willy is now more able to accept his fate, knowing now that it is a just one. And he is thankful for his fate because it has allowed him to now be accompanied in this painful and difficult life by his beloved wife from earlier lives. What would have been cause for despair and depression, namely the question, "Why do I have to bear this fate?" has now been clarified, making it unnecessary to become depressive and, in fact, giving cause for thankfulness: one may already clear up something in this life that would otherwise probably have been a barrier in one's next life.

And now his Higher Self revealed something else: his mother had also died at his birth for karmic reasons, because in earlier lives he had killed or taken mothers away from their children. And that was also the reason for his present feelings of guilt.

Now this statement is surely not easy to digest, meaning that his mother mainly had to die in order to make his karmic resolutions possible, i.e. he had to grow up without a mother's care. Also his mother's death in this life must therefore have been already planned for karmic reasons. Thus if we are born into a life without a mother's care and even with a terrible illness, and if all this – like everything else happening to us in life – is only aimed at helping us develop our inborn spirituality, then the persons and situations confronting us are only supporting actors and stage-props helping us reach our spiritual goal: to attain ever greater levels of love. And if, as we heard above, the body is not so important and the only real concern is mental and spiritual development, then we will have to re-think our whole previous way of thinking and considering human fates. We will need new ways of thinking concerning the reasons why we are here in this world.

But here I don't plan to begin such philosophizing, just to open new doors to the understanding of our being.

And now we shall come to the feet, in order to finish off our sampling of Regression Therapy "from head to foot".

26. The further effects of karmic bonds (ankles and wrists)

Karla is forty-seven years old. Because of massive fears she was put in a psychiatric hospital and forced to retire from her civil service job. The history of her illnesses is very extensive. At her first session I concentrated on freeing her from psychic pressures and from a curse hanging over her from earlier times. If possible, I also wanted to get to the bottom of her corpulence. A few weeks later she returned beaming with pleasure over the loss of fourteen pounds. She had also been freed of the disturbing extraneous influence that had bothered her for years. But now she also wanted to rid herself of pains in her feet, ankles, wrists and knees. She had already had to wear special insoles as a child because her feet hurt so much. Her ankles were weak. She felt as if she were bound at her hands and feet. These pains recurred often and seemed as if – I quote – "as if someone were saying to me, 'Look at me, do something!'"

The doctors could find nothing wrong. When she was a student – she was working half-days on the side – her knees hurt her so much that she believed herself to have rheumatism. She would often wake up crying – as she said – "like crazy from the pains". She often would cry in pain during the day. Between twenty and twenty-one her pains were the worst – then she could not even stand still.

The last doctor she visited could find nothing, just like so many other colleagues before, even accusing her of faking her pains to keep from having to work and study. (*So many people receive similar responses, although they really feel great pain.*) From that point she gave up seeking medical help – the doctors could find nothing no matter how hard they looked. (*Usually there is nothing concretely evident – these pains are not faked pains but karmic ones from earlier lives. In such cases the doctor should transfer his patient immediately to a regression therapist. Perhaps the latter can get to the bottom of these pains and eliminate them. In any case it will be necessary in the future for physicians and regression therapists to work together for the good of their patients. There is no way to avoid this.*)

In her life as a perpetrator she was a torturer named Franz in Germany in the year 1104 who not only dragged the people named to him by the authorities out of their houses and put them in prison iron-chained hand and foot, but also thought up special torture methods, e.g. crushing their feet. He took for himself whatever women or girls appealed to him.

In her life as a victim she was named Barbara, living in a hut as a twenty year-old French girl and healing others with herbs and oil. Because she was successful in healing, more and more people came to her. A married aristocrat, Henry, fell in love with her. Telling her that he was single, he succeeded in beginning a relationship with her. After it became public knowledge, his wife also confronted him with the news, threatening to have him punished for adultery, which would ruin his whole career. She demanded that he accused Barbara of witchcraft because she had seduced him, an otherwise faithful husband, by means of her magic arts. Intimidated by her threats, he accused Barbara of witchcraft, for which she has now been arrested and imprisoned.

A priest comes to her cell who she calls Frank and who

questions her, determined to make her confess to being a witch. This priest proves himself quickly to be a brutal sadist who is not even interested in her confession. In the presence of the guard he whips her until the clothes on her body are mere shreds. Then he orders her feet put in presses and the screws tightened, squashing her feet. When she still refuses to confess having bewitched Henry and having forced him to sleep with her, Frank takes a glowing iron and applies it to her stomach and knees. Then he has her wrists bound tighter and tighter with ropes. Finally he sends the torturers away and rapes the half-conscious woman.

For the next weeks he comes every day and tortures her as much as he wants. Every time he also rapes her. He has probably forbidden the guards to torture her more. He wants to do it all himself.

In the meantime she has become twenty-one years of age. Finally she is carried to the courtroom because she cannot walk any longer and is condemned to death by burning. On the day of her execution she is bound at her feet and arms to the stake, but before the flames can start to rise she curses Frank, the judges, the clergy, her torturers and the audience.

After her death she views the scene from above. Then two entities approach her who she calls angels. They take her before an apparently empty high chair that is surrounded by light. She believes it must be God's throne. There she hears telepathically a voice saying, "You had to burn because you also were a torturer and burned others." Suddenly she sees pictures in her mind from her life as the German torturer Franz.

Then she is led to small houses that, as she says, "glow".

There Barbara sees herself in a group of about sixteen souls being taught by a teacher, Philip. She remembers now having known him in earlier periods in the beyond. She is surprised that she can float or walk – whichever she likes at the moment. She even visits as a spirit the town again where she lived as Barbara.

Arriving at the Gate of Clouds, she hears that the wife of Henry is her present mother, with whom she, to put it mildly, has great problems. Henry is an acquaintance of hers who in various ways is quite interested in her, while Frank is her previous superior. A practitioner of black magic, Frank put pressure on her, finally mobbing her and driving her to a mental breakdown. The psychiatrist she sought help from then sent her to a mental hospital.

On the Mountain of Revelation she recognizes the karmic connections, accepts her life as a victim as Barbara as just punishment, offers the cup of love and reconciliation to all concerned and to herself in her lives as a perpetrator, as a victim and in her present life. Finally she takes the pinecone in her hand, stuffing it with all the things she has discovered and would like to free herself from. She says, "I hereby free myself from all my pains in my ankles and wrists, all pains in my feet, hands and knees. I free myself from the ugly skin on my stomach and knees (*which, as her Higher Self said, came from the burns through the glowing iron*), and I free myself from all my feelings of guilt."

Four months later she came to me once more to rid herself of further symptoms. She was in great spirits, saying, "After the last Regression Therapy session the pains in my joints disappeared gradually. After a week they had fully disappeared and they have never reappeared since." Then we began to work on her corpulence, a problem only briefly touched on in the first session. She was already convinced that this session would again be a full success.

One thing that is worth noting in the death as a witch described above is the fact that she was twenty when she entered the prison, was tortured and raped for several weeks, until she was twenty-one. This corresponds exactly to the age when she as Karla experienced the worst pains in her ankles, wrists, feet and knees. Here we see a phenomenon that often turns up in Regression Therapy, namely that tortures at a certain age in earlier lives will often turn up as bad pains in the present life at the very spots at the same age. As we see there is a karmic parallel in age, by which the body signals, "At this part of your body you have suffered something for karmic reasons. Discover what it is and free yourself from it."

We have unfortunately not yet had the opportunity to investigate all these lives in respect to the question if the pains in hands, feet, wrists, ankles and knees were always similar to those in the present life, or if they were perhaps missing in intermediate earth lives. Such research projects will be future themes for the doctoral dissertations of medical students. For the desire to approach such unexplored areas will inspire many scientifically oriented persons.

In all the above-mentioned cases of "somatic illnesses" it was seen that all the bodily symptoms could be led back to karmic causes. Thus all suffering through illness and the associated pains are based on karma. If the pains are major symptoms they constitute a balancing life as a victim; otherwise they may be seen as later repercussions of a life as a victim in which – because of previous lives as a perpetrator, of course – more or less terrible things were done to the body. Karma, karma, everywhere karma.

I could report still very many more treatments of symptoms and their balancing. For as a regression therapist I have – in contrast to many medical doctors – not specialized in certain restricted symptomatic fields. With every client who comes to me we can try together to find the causes and corresponding cures or solutions. But this book is only meant as an introduction to the existing possibilities respecting symptoms and their possible (or probable) elimination.

Now we want to turn to a very interesting area in Regression Therapy, namely the curing of karmic relationships, which is a special high light of Regression Therapy.

THE HEALING OF KARMIC RELATIONSHIPS

27. After the wedding: reappearing karmic patterns (Conflicts with one's husband)

Renata is a forty-nine year-old woman married to her husband Ulrich for twenty-six years. They have a daughter. After a few years of marriage Renata separated from her husband and moved to another town. And although they have not been intimate with each other since that time, Ulrich comes once in a while to visit, and he takes care of his wife and daughter financially. His presence is unbearable for her. Every mention of a coming visit – even if it is only to last one day – causes suffering for her even ahead of time. Although he is friendly and nice to her, she has the feeling that her chest is being squeezed in a vice. Nevertheless she is not able to bring herself to divorce him, although she has had new partners in the meantime (and still has). Something keeps her from final separation. She feels in his presence, as she says, like the rabbit in front of a snake. She is overcome by a feeling of helplessness and fear.

Chung I will call the five year-old boy (for she is not able to pronounce his real Chinese name) who lives in a palace in China. His father is very powerful and has a great number of wives. Chung's mother was a woman from far away, i.e. she was not Chinese. She was thrown out a few months ago and probably killed, so Chung does not know what really happened. He is told that she simply left. The five year-old is very sad and does not play any longer with his stepbrothers and stepsisters in the beautiful garden. His father is unapproachable and strict. Chung loves his mother more than everything and he is driven by the need to look for her. He takes advantage of his birthday celebration to have himself carried on a litter out of the palace. In the crowded streets he slips out of the litter and runs away. The four litter-bearers run after him, but he is able to hide. Though there is a great search made for him, he can remain undiscovered a few days. He sleeps on the ground, is hungry and cold. But one night, when he is very sad, he sees his mother before him. She looks like a shining apparition. She comforts him, covers him with his jacket and says, "I love you." But then the apparition disappears again.

A few days later Chung is discovered. He is brought before his father, who is very angry and orders his servant to whip him. After that his father orders something which he cannot understand. He is carried out and blinded so that he can never run away again. Chung now walks blinded with a cane through the garden. He wants to die. He feels helpless and is depressive. But then the contact to his mother within is successful. He can now communicate with her in thoughts. She soothes him and gives him courage to keep going. When he is eighteen enemies break into the palace. He hears the cries of the others, before a spear pierces his own breast. After death he sees his body below and is surprised that he can see again. Then he sees his mother. She hugs him and says, "I am proud of you."

At the Gate of Clouds Renata learns that the Chinese father who had her blinded is her present husband. In her life as a perpetrator she was a very large muscular man who was only called "the giant", who lived alone and was feared by all. Two courageous men approached him publicly and wanted to battle with him, thinking they were together stronger than him. The giant agreed to fight to the death with them without weapons. He grabbed one of them and put out his eyes with his fingers, causing the other to run away in fear. And as it turned out Renata's husband is the one who lost his eyesight through the giant. *(He wears glasses today. Perhaps his shortsightedness stems from that life.)*

Renata's soul was supposed to attain karmic resolution through the soul of her present husband by his having her blinded. (*It is not always true that the person who is injured fatally by someone is also the same one who carries out the karmic balancing event. It is rather the exception to the rule.*) Her life as the half-Chinese boy and the karmic events experienced there the following programming still had an effect on her present life: She was afraid to leave her husband and divorce him because she ran away from him in the earlier life and was punished by losing her sight. Subconsciously this program was still active, arousing the fear that he could again do something drastic to her. Her fear together with the tension felt in his presence resulted from her fear of the Chinese father. She felt as if in prison when he was near.

He knows subconsciously, on the other hand, that he has to make up to her for something. If they divorced, this possibility to rehabilitate himself would disappear. Therefore he, too, doesn't want a divorce, although this is for both sides only a pro-forma marriage. Their whole relationship is based on karmic grounds. Although the lives shown here represent only a small portion of the lives they have lived together in very different constellations, they are, especially the Chinese one, very revealing in respect to their mutual relationships.

But the question seems worth asking as to why Renata did not already feel this fear the first time she met her husband. Why did her tense feelings not turn up until a few years after her marriage? Because there are – as we have seen - no accidents, there must also be a fitting reason for this. Souls meet again and again until all their disharmonies are worked out, even if it takes hundreds of lives. (*Therefore to avoid having to meet a particular soul again in a later life one should clear up all the disharmonies in this life!*) When pairs are to meet again because disharmonies from earlier lives are still present, they are hit – like the ancient Romans would say – by Cupid's arrow of love, so that they decide to marry. Yes, apparently such pairs are somehow injected as well with a kind of "serum of forgetfulness" which temporarily covers up the problems to be worked on. The effect of this "serum" then gradually wears off, so that the old programs can come into effect again.

For Renata and her husband this "serum" was effective - up to the time their daughter was conceived. And the more the effect of the serum wore off, the more the old programs became obvious. Then the work could begin again (subconsciously) on clearing up the old unresolved behavior patterns, raising the questions, "Will there be progress this time or will the patterns become worse?" Sometimes this love-serum only lasts until the marriage-ceremony. How many spouses become aware at the moment of exchanging rings or while standing before the altar that this will be no harmonious marriage? Perhaps they will then be overcome by the fear of taking a false step. Or many may be aware of the danger of a bad marriage but at the same time feel subconsciously that for some unknown reason it is a step that must be taken. Such reasons can be brought to light by Regression Therapy, and, as we will see, the problems connected with them can be solved.

28. Our whole relationship is governed by karma (Conflicts with one's female partner)

Mario is in his middle thirties. He has been living with his partner Lisa for five years without marrying her – which up to now has not been so easy in Italy. They have together a three year-old son, and another child is on the way. Something prevents them from marrying formally, though both know that they belong together and will stay together.

Mario asked for this Regression Therapy session because he somehow feels bound to Lisa, although their relationship is constantly under stress and he is a good-looking man and would have no problem finding another partner. He can never satisfy her and is criticized constantly for not doing things properly, even if it is just hanging up a picture. She is always very critical and rational and takes life very seriously, while he sees everything as easy. Because he gives seminars and has to travel a lot, she thinks there is reason to believe that he is unfaithful. She complains constantly that he is never there and has no time for her and the family. But everything had begun so harmoniously. They could talk to each other about everything, especially esoteric subjects.

In the life revealed to him by his Higher Self as containing the main cause for their life together Mario recognizes himself as a twenty-seven year-old woman, Alina, in Switzerland around 1400. She is thinking about her father, Markus, for whom she feels sorry. He lives alone in the forest as a woodcutter. Now she reveals the background: Behind the back of her mother he began a sexual relationship with her at the age of thirteen. This was carried out whenever the mother left the house for several hours. One day, when Alina was seventeen, the mother returned unexpectedly and discovered them together in bed. The mother ran screaming out of the house into the fields. Two days later she hanged herself.

Then the daughter decided to stop the relationship with her father. The father, full of guilt, was despondent. She was afraid that he, too, would commit suicide. Her father then started crying and pleading with the daughter, saying she would have now more than ever to replace her mother and shouldn't refuse him. But she stuck to her decision.

Her father then became more emphatic, claiming that she was his property because he had conceived her and that it was his right to do what he wanted with her. And because his daughter didn't have the strength or courage to leave him – where could she go with the dangers waiting everywhere for a young, single girl – she finally decided to stay. In the long run she also could not refuse herself to him sexually. So they remained on the road to destruction: at twenty-five she became pregnant. The worst had thus come to pass. She wanted to bear the child at any cost, but he was aware of the consequences – incest being a mortal sin, punishable by death or at least a long prison sentence. He obtained an abortion medicine, which proved to be successful.

After she had recovered, she summoned all her courage and left him. But later her thoughts often wandered to him. At the age of thirty-five she visited him again in the forest to see how he was doing. He was extremely depressive but surprised and happy to see his lover-daughter again. She was awfully sorry for him, but determined to leave him again nevertheless. He tried desperately to convince her to stay, maintaining his right as the father to determine the life of his unmarried daughter. Seeing that he could not sway her mind, he pulled a knife in desperation and threatened her. She defended herself, and in the tussle he fell over, jabbing the knife in his own stomach. He moaned and died. Alina, not knowing what to do, ran away. She felt afraid but at the same time liberated. Later she married but remained childless. She died as a widow at the age of sixty-six in Aar. Her "never-again" sentence: "I will never again lose a child."

After death she hovers over her body, while neighbors are approaching it. She meets her mother and also her father again in the beyond. Both appear younger and more attractive than ever. She does not criticize her father. Then she meets a small child and realizes suddenly that it is her own aborted child. *This requires an explanation. In the beyond, time as we know it doesn't exist. If one has died as a child, one can remain many "years" in this form, grow older or (immediately) take the form of an adult. Or for special reasons one may take again the form of a child after already being an adult. Here the soul of the aborted baby takes again the form of a child, because his mother had wished for one all her life.*

All four of them belong to a group of souls, twelve of whom are present (*some members of the group are incarnated and thus not present at the moment, though they are being taken care of invisibly, wherever they may be*). She meets her leader in the beyond whose name is Gabriel. (*This is not the Archangel Gabriel. Many soul-guides like to adopt the names of archangels or saints.*) Alina learns from two of the helpers assigned to this group, a man and a woman, why she had to have all these terrible experiences with her father on earth. As a man, she had also misused her father, who was then her daughter. She had to experience what it is like to be forced as a daughter to cohabit with one's father. She needed this experience in order to grow in love. The aborted child had been married to the father in a still earlier life, when Alina was a young wanderer who raped her while he was away.

Arriving again at the Gate of Clouds, Mario learns from his Higher Self that his present son is the mother of Alina, that the aborted child is now Lisa's child-to-be and that the former father is his present partner, Lisa. Both of them have received in this life the opportunity to raise the two children and give them all the love that was missing before. Beyond this there was only one life in which he had been closely associated with Lisa.

Their present life is determined by karmic factors. Their present behavior toward their present child and their coming child is marked by great care. For they subconsciously wish to make up to these children for past abuses. Above all they will show especially great care for the second child, which had previously been aborted. The first child will carry the thought-patterns of the previous mother who had hanged herself. It will surely often be stubborn, have its feelings hurt and reproach its parents. Perhaps it will even be unexplainably envious of its own present mother. Of course, it will also have problems with its present father, having been cheated as his previous wife when he misused her own daughter.

As we can see, all of our relationships are conditioned by karmic feelings, attitudes and behavioral patterns from earlier lives. For the patterns acquired in earlier lives have been carried over from one life to the next, gradually being modified by more harmonious feelings and experiences. We could also speak of a very interesting interpersonal "game" spread over many lives. In the beyond we "take a break" so-to-speak, where the seriousness and passion of the game itself is interrupted. As we have seen, Alina's mother and father and even the aborted child spent the time in the beyond in harmony with one another.

Of course, there are also those who are so involved in the "game" that in their minds they even keep on playing passionately after the "referee's whistle", i.e. death, especially if the latter came unexpectedly. Perhaps they stay on earth (as ghosts) or create artificial worlds like the "dark spheres" mentioned earlier (where they carry on further their habitual patterns of thoughts, feelings and actions).

But sooner or later we go back to our "game" on the earthly playing field. Whoever finally becomes completely loving, after many earthly lives, is the "winner". But actually everyone will be the winner sooner or later, as the Higher Intelligence has arranged for everyone to win at some time. Actually we are all already winners and have finished many games on other playing fields but have decided to enter into a new game on the planet earth, where we now find ourselves.

The fact that Mario and Lisa live together without yet wanting to officially marry has to do with the fact that in their earlier life as father and daughter they lived together as a pair, knowing "we cannot and dare not be publicly a pair." This program still affects subconsciously their relationship, which is also still burdened by feelings of guilt.

Lisa, the previous father, is determined to make for his misdeeds to Alina, the previously abused daughter. Nonetheless, she takes the more masculine part, while Mario plays more the feminine role. This is logical from the karmic point of view. And Alina, who always wanted to leave her father, plays this part today as Mario, who regularly leaves Lisa, as the previous father, and returns again.

We carry on our behavioral patterns from earlier lives, even though the different roles may be differently distributed. Markus, the previous father, is now Lisa, i.e. a woman; Alina is presently Mario. A reincarnation expert can judge from the family constellations what the previous interrelationships may have been. For present family members were generally already bound together by family bonds in earlier lives.

These are exciting games, and they are supposed to be that way. For the more exciting they are, the more we involve ourselves in them through our feelings, thoughts and deeds. By being actively and intensively involved we learn also the most from these games. We also learn from our mistakes, which we can correct again in the next round. What a wonderful sport! For at the end everyone wins! Everyone will reach the end and be a winner in unconditional love. Who thought this sport up? Surely a grand master, someone many would name "God".

Whoever has already understood this sport and already is able and willing to love unconditionally is already a winner.

And I have the feeling that Mario will already be a winner in this life, for he is now learning Regression Therapy and gaining a deep comprehension of the secrets of the sport of life.

29. When karma is negative on both sides (Conflicts between mother and daughter)

Anna is a middle-aged, but still very active physician. She has had great problems with her mother almost all her life. They have rejected each other totally, and Anna is even afraid of her mother, who is now 80 years old. She has also a tense relationship with her father, feeling herself to be humiliated, forced and suppressed. She was always aware of the fact that she was rejected by her mother in favor of her two sisters and younger brother.

Every psychologist would now say, "She certainly only studied medicine to show her parents: 'You have all misunderstood me. Despite this I have reached a high goal. You should actually be proud of me and see that I should be your dearest child. You should be ashamed of giving me no or too little love as a child.'"

After I had put Anna in the alpha-state, we asked her Higher Self to show us where this life – beginning as a fetus – contained causes for the mutual rejection of mother and daughter. I asked if she was present at her conception, knowing from Regression Therapy sessions that souls sometimes want to be present there in order to experience practically the engendering of the body they will later occupy.

In fact she observes her parents already as newly-weds. They married three weeks ago and are skiing now in the mountains. In their room there are two single beds, but the husband finally slips into the bed of his wife, who reacts negatively, saying, "Not now already." Anna then sees that her mother soon begins to have bodily disturbances. She goes to her doctor (*Anna knew the doctor's name suddenly: Dr. Zimmermann.*), who reveals to her that she is pregnant. The mother, who feels herself not yet ready to have a child, says, "Well, if it has to be." The father is happy about the news, but the mother remains ambivalent.

Nevertheless Anna now goes into the fetus. From the third month on the mother begins to feel Anna's vibrations and gets abdominal pains. She doesn't want the child at all any more and hopes to have an abortion. Anna now senses her mother's rejection. This fact alone is enough to produce later a negative attitude on the part of the daughter, expressing itself in hate, fear and/or an inferiority complex. As Anna further relates in trance, she nearly suffocates during birth.

Now we go from one important event to the next: While being breast-fed her head is held so tightly that she nearly suffocates. Her mother is not at all gentle with her. While putting on her diapers her mother screams at her daughter, asking why she couldn't have had her toilet before. And crying once when her head gets stuck in the side of the crib, she is thrown on her back by her mother, who grabs her around the neck and shakes her, saying, "You stupid Anna!"

Whenever her mother screams at her, Anna tries to hide out of fear. But when she is sad, she sees a light at her bedside and hears a voice telling her, "You see, you are not alone." (*It seems to me that mothers or others would be more careful in many respects if they knew that everything one does or says to someone else remains stored in their subconscious and can, e.g. in Regression Therapy, be brought back to consciousness. For those in the beyond, however, everything is visible. Nothing that happens on earth or is said or done there will be kept secret – unless out of the desire for discretion.*)

At the age of three, Anna is discovered by her mother as she is apparently playing with her clitoris. She looks at her with contempt and says, "You mustn't do that. That is awful!" (*We can see how prudish certain societies still are today. Or does it have to do with oneself?*) She gives her "misbehaving" daughter a slap and scolds her while dressing her, adding her favorite remark, "You stupid Anna!" Her mother never hugs her, and when her father gives her a kiss on the forehead, her mother turns away ostentatiously. When she is three, her mother tells her, "I don't want you." When Anna is eight, she is proud of her braids, but her mother hates them. She braids Anna's hair only with distaste, so that Anna sometimes cries out of pain. One day her mother says, "I am tired of plaiting your braids." She grabs her arm, drags her crying to the hairstylist and has them cut off. For Anna the loss of the braids is like the loss of her head, and she cries a long time afterwards.

When Anna at ten sees her mother kissing her little brother while carrying him on her arm, she asks her mother which of them she likes best. Her mother looks at her almost hatefully, saying, "Don't act so stupid, you dumb thing!"

The reader might ask himself why I go so extensively into her present childhood and her relationship to her mother. But we shall see that their relationship can be traced back to karmic programming.

Arriving again at the Gate of Clouds, we ask her Higher Self to lead Anna into an earlier life where her soul met her present mother and which is important for their problematical relationship. Suddenly she was a nineteen year-old knight named Heinrich von Zurlinden, to whom his lord, a powerful knight named von Muralt, had given a letter meant for the latter's beloved, the daughter of his enemy, Count Hans Konrad. His was the dangerous mission to take the letter to the castle and give it to her secretly without being caught.

The young knight understands the danger, but at the castle he is interrogated and searched, and the letter is found. He is thrown into the dungeon, where he is treated callously.

There is another man in prison there, a flour-thief, who says, "You will never leave here." But the next day he is dragged out again. The master of the castle is there, together with his executioner, who is carrying a sword. Heinrich bows down and says, "Please don't do anything to me, I was just delivering the letter." He is then dragged onto the scaffold. Other inhabitants of the castle have gathered around and are jeering. Hans Konrad gives the executioner the sign. Heinrich is pulled to his knees. He cries, "No!" but then he is already beheaded. (*If there are authors lacking historical material for their novels, I would recommend to them to collect it in bushels as regression therapists!*)

Suddenly he sees himself in a wonderful area. An "angel" (*the unexperienced often take the entities in the beyond for angels*) greets him. Other entities gather. He is bathed, and his neck is treated and healed. Finally he is led to a court of judges in blue gowns. He is supposed to say what he thinks of his life and activities on earth. The judges, sometimes laughing in a friendly way, say that he has been very naïve. Then he visits his parents on earth as a spirit to console them for the loss of their son and to tell them how nicely he is being treated. (*Many of the dead return to their mourners, trying to comfort them. Sometimes they are even noticed in one way or another.*) From her Higher Self Anna learns that Count Hans Konrad is her present mother.

In the next life Anna discovers herself as a kind of aborigine named Oala. He is running, spear in hand, after a man into whose back he then throws the spear. The man is mortally wounded, and Oala is proud of this at first, saying, "I just wanted to see if I could hit him." The man belonged to another tribe, but they were not at war. The head of the tribe orders him to appear before him and scolds him for his "stupid" act. Firstly, it was cowardly to kill someone from behind, and, secondly, they would now have war with the other tribe. The chief throws him out of the tribe for his cowardice and stupidity (!). He has to leave behind all his possessions and live alone in the wilderness. He becomes remorseful, regretting his stupid act. He dies alone fourteen years later.

After death, a shining entity appears, leading him under a green waterfall. It then offers him a pink cape, saying, "This will help you to overcome your sadness." But he is also reminded of other bad deeds. For example he strangled another man. He must now stay under a roof of leaves at another place until he also feels regret for that deed.

Finally he is led before a court of three men in blue robes. There are three other men there who also were murderers in their earthly lives. And one of the judges says to him, "You knew that you are not allowed to kill. You are not allowed to judge over the lives of others." Furthermore, he is told that once for every murder carried out on earth he will have to reincarnate and experience the same fate. And he accepts that as just. As perpetrators we are also led by others in the beyond – after experiencing regret – to recognize that very knowledge which we actually already had within ourselves but which was covered over by our ego: the knowledge that the same or similar deeds that we have committed against others out of lovelessness and callousness will at some time also have to be committed against us. As soon as we have realized this – under the guidance perhaps of previous friends, relatives, family members, spirit-guides, teachers or even angels – we can easily accept this law of karma and are willing to condemn ourselves or allow ourselves to be condemned to the same fate.

Before the Gate of Clouds Anna hears that the man who was previously killed from behind is her present brother. The chief who threw him out of the tribe because of stupidity (!) is her present mother. This has probably led to her present standard phrase for her daughter: "You are a stupid Anna!"

The life as Oala preceded the life as Heinrich von Zurlinden. Thus the life in which he was beheaded was a karmic life resulting from that of Oala. But he was also a farmer who had to fight in Switzerland against the Austrians in 1386. He was armed with a spear and placed in the front battle-line by his leader, who didn't like him. This being practically his death-sentence, he died of a neck-wound inflicted by another soldier's lance.

And again he stands before the judges in blue robes. This time they say, "You have acted rightly." They want to express that he has now made up for his deeds as Oala. But there are still other deeds of callousness to balance. So Anna is ready to balance them in the coming life.

She recognizes herself suddenly as a seventeen year-old young Red Indian man named Igall. He is strong and courageous and is to receive the special honor of being offered to the gods. His people has been taught to see this as the highest goal of life and of utmost importance in satisfying the gods. He accepts this honor gladly, although with some private queasiness. His head is then separated from the body.

In the beyond he again meets the three judges in blue, who praise him for carrying out this task well and without rebelling. But he also hears that the gods to whom he was offered were not really gods but a fiction. "You always desire a test. You think you are a hero. But there is still too much pride in you, so you have to learn humility." And the judges say that he has to be reborn as a woman who loses her child and then also her husband in war and then has to live as a beggar for the rest of her life. This is necessary for him to learn humility. He would however now have a free choice of his parents in the chosen country as well as of whatever nice things he would like to experience there. So this soul chooses for the first twenty-four years a nice, happy life. For he knows that the following years on earth will be years of hard testing.

According to the philosopher Pythagoras[36] three different types of souls enter into the beyond. The first type includes those who were callous and inconsiderate when they were on earth. They are given their next lives on earth as victims. The second group is made up of those who have done good as well as bad deeds. For them the next life is partially pre-determined, but they are also allowed to choose many things that they would like to experience or learn. The third group contains those who have done many good things in their previous lives but still have some things to learn or to balance. They are allowed to arrange their coming life themselves out of higher insight and knowledge.

The soul of Anna is to be counted among the second

---

36. Schuré, p. 300

group. The law of karma is understood and accepted by all the souls, irregardless of the group to which they belong. But choice and arrangement regarding one's next life is only possible to a limited extent – unless one is already counted among the more advanced souls. (*It is shameful to see how the great knowledge of such a wise man as Pythagoras could have been ignored in human philosophy, although it has finally been proved correct by Regression Therapy!*)

At the Gate of Clouds Anna learns that the priest who cut her head off is her present mother. Furthermore, as her Higher Self says, Anna herself has chosen her as a mother for her present life in order to learn to love her.

This is a hard statement! She could think, "To have to learn to love someone who has cut my head off in the previous life, who already had me decapitated as a young knight, who sent me (as Oala) into the lonely wilderness and put me (as a Swiss soldier) intentionally in the front line! And I am supposed to love my present mother, who has already caused me so many pains and troubles in life and who I have learned to hate from the core of my existence? My mother is already eighty years old, so there is not much time left to make up for things left undone."

For what one has failed to do in this life will be carried over to one's next life or later lives. Therefore her resolution formula after passing the cup is: "I free myself from my naivety, rashness, pride and from the rejection and fear of my mother." It is never too late to resolve a karmic debt with someone, even if the person is already in a coma or has even already died. If the person is dead, then the request for forgiveness can be received on a psychic level. But if one still has the opportunity of reaching the person in a fully conscious state, it is better to take advantage of this and not to wait until after death. This is true irregardless of whether forgiveness is to be requested or to be given – or both, as would be justified in this case.

And the effect of such resolution will be the subject of the next report.

30. Karmic balancing after eleven lives (Disharmonic relationships with one's mother and wife)

Michael is in his late forties and living in his third marriage with his wife Britta. From his first marriage he has one child, from the second two, whereas the third marriage will probably remain childless. He met Britta three years ago, and they decided to marry after three-quarters of a year. But just after the wedding her interest in sex began to lessen. Finally she refused to have any sex. Now any kind of intimacy, even hugging is unpleasant for her.

Michael grew up with his mother as an only child. When he was four, his father left. His mother was very strict with her son and, as he says, often "beat him verbally". At the age of twenty he finally escaped from her clutches by moving out. Even today they have no heartfelt relationship. He didn't see his father until much later – and then only met him rarely, until also this contact faded away. Michael suffers from a great number of symptoms: various allergies as well as bronchial congestion. He was cross-eyed as a child, which was relieved by operation. In front of a crowd he cannot speak a word. As soon as there are a number of persons speaking, his ability to hear almost disappears. His mother had him fostered once as a child, to which he attributes his fear of loss. In an earlier Regression Therapy session he had experienced himself jabbing someone in the foot with a lance, for which reason he had to live in a balancing life as a victim as a thief in Turkey whose feet were broken as a punishment. Michael has already had several professions, but is interested in becoming a faith healer, for which he has now had himself trained.

In this Regression Therapy session Michael wanted to find out why he had had so much trouble with his mother and also with Britta, his third wife, and why these two also dislike each other.

The first life into which his Higher Self then led him was one in Egypt in 1610 A.D. His name was Jonas. He was a Christian (a Coptik?) and worked as a faith healer. He can even see into bodies and cure inner illnesses with mental energy. Sick people are carried to him and can walk home on their own two legs. He connects himself, as he says, with God and His love, letting this energy flow through his hands. Therefore many people come to him for help, and he quickly becomes a popular healer.

His marriage with Martia was arranged. She is never satisfied, and her provocative manner often makes him react aggressively. They live together at the house of Jonas' mother, with whom Martia is constantly fighting, for which reason Jonas criticizes his wife. She wanted to have a child, but seems to be infertile. Now she orders him to drive away all his other patients and apply all his healing powers to her. In an attack of rage he stabs her to death, for which he is hanged.

After death he feels immediate relief, meeting later a white-haired spirit-guide or teacher dressed in a turquoise robe who calls himself Moses. Moses discusses the spiritual laws with Jonas, saying, "Everything good or bad that you do returns to you. In the same way that you killed you were also killed yourself." Jonas knows this spiritual law, for he had also occupied himself with secret knowledge. Therefore he sees his death as justified. He is made aware that he has done a lot of good deeds, but that he still must learn to control his anger. He should have shown Martia the same love that he was always willing to give to others.

At the Gate of Clouds Michael learns from his Higher Self that his previous beloved mother is his present wife and his previous wife, Martia, is his present mother. They haven't learn to like each other yet. His present mother is also still subconsciously resentful to him for various reasons, so she treated him badly as a child. In this life he also receives from Britta no love, having refused it to Martia previously. And the wish to regain his previous healing is countered by the answer that he will have also to re-establish his connection to God.

Since we had now learned something about Michael's mother, now his wife, we asked his Higher Self to reveal to us other reasons why Michael was rejected by her in bed.

He sees himself suddenly as a king's son in Rumania. His name is Ramosch, and at the age of twenty-four he is already a war leader. He is courageous and strong and has proved himself to be something of a daredevil in battle. Now he has fallen in love with a twenty year-old aristocratic woman named Sentia. He breaks into her chamber. Rejecting him, she asks him to leave. Although he assures her of his love, she remains adamant. He refuses to go and grabs her, tears off her clothes and throws her on her bed. When she cries for help, he holds her mouth and rapes her.

She leaves the court for unknown parts, while Ramosch throws himself into battle again, beheading many warriors with his axe and raping other women now and again at will. He boasts to his soldiers that he can get any woman. And soon he meets a woman, Erra, who he falls in love with and who seems to return his affections. When she, however, doesn't immediately respond to his stormy advances, he whips her with his belt and rapes her. And again she leaves him.

But this woman he cannot forget, knowing that his wild manner destroyed the budding love they felt for one another. He becomes aware of all his misdeeds: He has killed many persons or had them killed, has tortured many or had them tortured. He has violated many women with no consideration for their feelings.

His conscience begins to torture him more and more. He becomes afraid of God's punishment. At the age of forty-nine he joins a monastery after confessing all of his sins to his father confessor and transferring the rule to one of his sons. At the age of sixty-four Ramosch dies.

After death he sees his body lying on the bed in his cell. He suddenly feels free. Monks come, stand around his body and pray for his soul. Then his body is placed in a casket. He experiences his own funeral in complete detail, for he floats over his grave and is surprised to read the thoughts of all the monks. I ask him what he in respect to his life would never do again. He answers spontaneously, "I will never kill again, never rape women and never misuse my power."

In the beyond he finds himself finally in a group of ten to twelve souls who he recognizes as "familiar faces" from earlier lives or periods in the beyond. They are led by a teacher named Johannes, wearing a light-blue toga. The other members of the group wear robes of various colors, his own being yellow.

All of them are occupied at the moment with his life as Ramosch. He re-lives it in thoughts, and the others can also experience it at the same time. He sees himself killing and raping. The others do not condemn him for his deeds, but they recognize his mistakes and speak about them. Ramosch is overcome by pain and sorrow over his misdeeds, none of which is hidden from the other members of the group. He feels ashamed and is ready and willing to resolve his deeds by suffering himself what he caused others. He has raped twenty-two women in all. He will have to meet these persons until all the things standing in the way of their reconciliation are rebalanced by love. So he has something to make up for to them all.

The law of karma is discussed in great detail. All present see it as just. Ramosch gradually prepares himself for a new life in which a part of what he has done to others will now be done to him. In this way the further development of his soul will be advanced by appropriate equalizing experiences. (*The great regret for his deeds that he had already experienced in the monastery will certainly have shortened his period in the preparatory purgatory – a time previous to the present group meeting.*)

Without returning to the Gate of Clouds and his Higher Self, I led Michael immediately into the life for which Ramosch had now prepared himself. We went directly to a very important experience for him. He sees himself now as a woman of the lowest aristocratic class at a ball in France. She hears the music (*sometimes I let them hum a few bars of the music*) in the ballroom, which is wonderfully illuminated by candlelight. Her name is Marie-Therese and she is longing to meet the man of her lifetime, if possible someone from the upper aristocracy. And such a man is constantly courting her. His name is Marbert. He is a member of one of the best families and rich, but she doesn't find him attractive. By saying that he wants to drink and speak to her alone, he does manage to get her into a private booth, where he reveals himself as a wolfish rascal. He forces her onto the couch. She tries to defend herself but cannot withstand his strength. She cries for help, but the music is too loud. She feels pain as he enters her. Finally he leaves her lying there. She feels herself humiliated and abused as a piece of goods for the pleasure of the higher aristocracy.

Later she also makes the mistake of telling her girl friends about it. Though they find it hard to believe, one of them spreads the gossip. Finally it reaches the ears of the lord of the castle, who causes Marie-Therese to be banned from the court as a liar. She is angry about this injustice and feels at the same time sadness. She liked the life at court and had felt so sure about eventually finding the right husband there. She becomes a market merchant, lies with men whenever she pleases, sometimes taking money for it, and is occasionally raped. At thirty-four she marries a blacksmith with whom she has three children. At fifty-four she dies.

After leading Michael back to the Gate of Clouds, I ask him what title he would give to this life. He answers, "The Resolution," meaning that this life was a part of the balancing events necessary to clear up what he had done as Ramosch. (*But that was only the resolution – or part of it – for what he had done as Ramosch to Sentia. For he will certainly have to meet Erra, too, in one or more later lives in order to make up something there. Then there are also others whom he had raped. Thus it is easy to understand that one life as a perpetrator may draw many balancing lives in its wake.*)

From his Higher Self Michael learns now that that Sentia in the life as Ramosch is his present Britta. Marbert, who ruined Marie-Therese, is his oldest son, already a dialysis patient as a teenager. The life as Ramosch took place around 900 A.D., and from this life about thirty-two follow-up lives have taken place up to the present date to make up for some of his misdeeds (*In some of them he also surely died in childhood.*) In his life as Marie-Therese he was raped seventeen times, while the other five rapes to be balanced out were spread out among his other lives as a woman. Britta rejected him in bed because she had been raped by him as Sentia, but she had also had similar experiences with men in other lives.

They had already spent eleven lives together since the life as Sentia and Ramosch (their first together) in order to learn from each other. He was asked to be understanding and patient with her. And he should ask her for forgiveness for what happened then. (This was done with the offering of the golden cup.) They had met in the beyond and had decided to balance out in this life the rest of the karmic debts between them. It had been suggested by the members of his group in the beyond, of which she was also a member, that they should meet in this life to finally "close the books" on this chapter.

But in the present life Michael was to first be together with two other women to settle some debts with them and/or to learn something. And these learning processes are not yet finished. A little is still missing, although Michael has had a total of 449 earthly lives, of which about 200 were masculine.

It could again be asked why Britta's dislike of Michael wasn't already apparent before their marriage. They had liked each other very much in the group in the beyond and this sympathy was re-established in this life until the time of their wedding. *This is another very interesting question, a variation of the "arrow of Cupid" that I spoke about in Case 27. It is clarified here that feelings of temporary attraction based perhaps on an attraction in the beyond may last for a while in one's relationship. Nevertheless we may finally reject this harmony in accordance with older underlying patterns of mutual distaste that have to be resolved in a deeper way and through a new reconciliation. Finally this should lead to a harmonious partnership and, ultimately, harmony on earth. Such a process can of course take many earth-lives. And as one can see from this, karma offers us the way to overcome many barriers and finally arrive at our goal: LOVE.*

Finally Michael offers all the main persons in this process the golden cup of love and reconciliation, the cup of resolution of suffering and guilt. Then he offers it to himself, saying, "I free myself of callousness, hate, dishonesty, scolding, self-doubt, all my fears, insecurity, guilt-feelings, vacillation, pressures, and I free myself of the disharmony in my relationship with Britta and my mother."

One can learn in a Regression Therapy session - from the Higher Self, from a entity in the beyond or through personal insight on the Mountain of Revelation – why one has sought out a particular partner (i.e. what the partners have to balance out or learn from one another). Then one knows the meaning of the particular partnership and can forgive more easily. Understanding why the other person acts (or has to act) in a certain way, one doesn't always immediately think of divorce or separation when disturbances arise. All of a sudden everything, or at least almost everything, becomes clear. Where previously there was fogginess or even chaos within and without, suddenly meaning and insight, understanding and forgiveness appear – as possible precursors of renewed attraction and love.

For everything has a meaning. Every one of us has sought out our partner for a very special reason. Only when the reason has been fulfilled can we part again. But to do this the reason must be understood first. Regression Therapy offers this possibility of understanding.

I believe that in this new millennium we can learn to investigate all our karmic relationships and live them more effectively. Then we will succeed in eliminating them for good from our karmic freight, so that for our next life we no longer need choose certain persons, i.e. our "team-members", out of karmic necessity but just in order to live together harmoniously on earth with them.

About half a year later I phoned Michael to find out about possible improvements in his relationships with his mother and his wife. And he stated that those relationships indeed improved tremendously.

31. When karma suddenly ends (Complete rejection by one's mother)

Manuela is a beautician who has made her aim not only to beautify the outward appearance of people but also to kindle their "inner flame". Thus she has supplemented her beauty farm also with a bookstore. In the latter there is not only literature to expand one's consciousness and quality of life but also many decorative things from gems over glittering mobiles, Aurosoma bottles, Bach flower essences down to special aroma-essences for inner and outer well-being. She is divorced, in her middle forties and has a daughter.

As a participant in one of my training seminars she wanted to know why she was so strongly rejected by her mother[37] who had already had problems during pregnancy. The fetus caused her increasing bodily pains and the birth was very difficult. After Manuela had finally seen the light

37. Manuelas story was already related in condensed form in my book *Rebirth- the evidence.*

of day and had been cleaned and given to her mother to breast-feed, she was unwilling to touch her and never did breast-feed her.

Her whole childhood became a torture, as her mother could not even stand her being in the same room but sent her out immediately or just ignored her. So she learned early in life to avoid her mother as much as possible. Never was she touched or stroked or even given any kind of pleasant comment. She could see how her mother touched or stroked her other children and called them by baby-names. But towards Manuela her attitude was completely different.

Finally Manuela was able to leave her parent's house at seventeen. Her mother never even called her up. But when she had a child of her own, she felt obligated to sometimes take it to see its grandparents. Such an event was Christmas, when she brought her little daughter together with a present for the grandparents to their house. While her daughter was inside the living room singing carols under the lit Christmas Tree with the rest of the family, Manuela had to wait outside in the hall because her mother could not stand her in the same room.

This was Manuela's story, related in the alpha-state in front of the group of Regression Therapy trainees: She saw herself suddenly as a young and very beautiful woman in bourgeois Vienna around 1770. I'll name her Constance. She was having a very intensive secret affair with an influential man. They were in love with each other and would certainly have married, if the man had not already had a wife. In those days marriage was considered a God-given sacrament. Adultery was an affront for God and could be punished by being sent to hell or other unpleasant sanctions. Thus a divorce was out of the question. A public scandal would also have endangered her lover's influential position and further career.

In such cases there was only one proven but infamous means: one had to "eliminate" the barrier to a new marriage. After Constance had succeeded in poisoning the wife of her lover, nothing stood in the way of a new public marriage.

At the Gate of Clouds Manuela learns that the woman poisoned by her then is now her mother. Now it is obvious to her why her mother rejected her from the beginning, not even wanting the fetus in her womb.

To all those taking part in the seminar it was already clear that every soul emits totally individual vibrations recognizable by other souls that it comes in contact with. The emotional body of the woman she poisoned had registered Constance's vibrations as those of her murderer. The emotional body is carried from incarnation to incarnation until all the negative programs contained in it have been totally erased. Thus the vibrations had been carried over into the life of her mother, influencing her mother to want to reject the fetus after Constance's soul had entered into it and subsequently made this pregnancy a nightmare for her.

Now Constance could understand why her mother didn't want to be anywhere near her – she was psychically "allergic" to her! The whole range of reactions of her mother was thus explainable on the basis of karma, making it now easy for her to offer her the cup of love and reconciliation. First she goes into her life as Constance, offering it to the wife of her lover and expressing her heartfelt wish for forgiveness. Then she visualizes herself going to her present mother, standing before her, offering her also the cup, asking her for forgiveness for the offenses she had committed and finally offering the cup to herself, thus freeing herself from all her guilt.

A week later she reported the following events to me: "You will not believe it. Returning home from the seminar, I had just entered the house and still had my hand on the doorknob when the telephone rang. I just managed to reach it. Just guess who was on the other end! My mother! It was the first phone-call I had ever received from her in my whole life! And she said, 'My Love....', that was the very first time she had ever called me that, 'I know that you would like to travel next summer to America. By chance (!) an American is visiting me tomorrow afternoon. Do come tomorrow for tea at four o'clock so I can introduce this gentleman to you. He can surely give you a lot of information.'" Speechless at first, Manuela then agreed to go. But she could not understand what had suddenly come over her mother? She asked herself, "Could it possibly have been the reincarnation session?"

The next day Manuela rang at four p.m. at the door of her parents' house. Opening the door for her, her mother gave her a heartfelt hug and led her by the hand to meet the guest. Her mother's previous rejection had experienced a 180° turnaround. Three years later, after Manuela had already become herself a very successful regression therapist, I met her at a congress. I asked her how her relationship to her mother had been developing, to which she answered, "We have become good friends."

What had happened? The soul of the poisoned woman, who was now present in the body of Manuela's mother, had waited almost 250 years in the hope that the soul of her murderer would apologize. And after this had taken place, the rejection of her daughter disappeared. In other words, the negative karmic band between mother and daughter was suddenly broken and existed no longer. Another thing that is remarkable is that this process took place in the seminar-room, i.e. far away from her mother's house. Nevertheless her mother somehow took note of the apology and subconsciously accepted it, although she was never consciously informed of it.

We humans are still very ignorant in respect to the many secret processes controlling our mutual attraction and repulsion. We are aware of the laws of transmission of physical waves, but we know almost nothing of the laws of transmission or transfer of psychic waves. We still have a great number of things to learn, also in areas that we presently do not take seriously – areas that we may need humility and courage to enter into.

It is interesting to note in this example the intervention of invisible powers, which were most certainly responsible for this karmic resolution process. They must have arranged for the mother to invite an American to tea, offering a perfect opportunity for reconciliation at just the right time. Even stranger seems the fact that her mother hugged her at the doorstep, as if there had never been any differences between them. This reconciliation had certainly been agreed upon previously in the beyond between Manuela's soul and that of her mother.

Certainly it will not always be so easy to resolve disharmonious karmic relationships and change them into harmonious ones. But if Regression Therapy allows us to delve into the basic karmic processes, which cause disharmony in relations, and in many cases to heal the resulting wounds, this in itself will be a blessing for mankind and one of the greatest achievements with which we can face the new millennium.

Part Four

The Concept of Karma in a Modern Light

In the All-Oneness the free choice of karmic reactions is made

Haven't I chosen my fates since creation myself?

(Novalis)

To investigate the real meaning of reincarnation and karma we will have to widen our scope and inquire into their meaning within the higher plan of existence. Our questions are: "Where do we come from?" "What does it look like there?" "Why have we entered into this journey of the soul through many lives?" And a common denominator to all these questions has resulted from our many investigations in the alpha-state into the lives of different persons, taking them back to the origin of their being, there where everything began.

If we can trust what the human subconscious reveals in the alpha-state – and the successes of Regression Therapy lead us to believe that we can – then another chapter in the history of the development of humanity may open up, a chapter that in contrast to other chapters is not based on speculation and belief, but is open to empirical testing – namely by returning in Regression to the source of all existence.

Those in trance have attempted to describe this source of all existence. Drawing on these descriptions, I will try to give the reader at least an approximate impression in words of that which actually defies all description: Everything is spirit. Everything is oneness. Everything is bliss. Everything is love. One needs no thinking, no feelings, and no forms. And at the same time one is potentially everything. This state can be described as "Being God". There are no differences in this All-Oneness. Everything is one.

As far as I know, in Western thought only Plotinus has come close to understanding this, based on the four enlightenment experiences that he again and again tries to describe. But in other places, above all in India, other enlightened persons have had the opportunity to experience this unity briefly – often only for a fraction of a second – describing this almost indescribable state as oneness with God.

Everything there is in harmony. There is neither space nor time, but there is an inexhaustible supply of imaginative power, which can be activated as desired. If one wishes, one can imagine oneself as one or many parts of this All-Oneness - or as one part dividing itself into unlimited tiny parts. Nevertheless one remains always in the oneness. One can so-to-speak "play games" with one's imagination, creating one's own space and time perceptions and even imagining oneself there in a form with body, feelings and mental powers. In this unity or All-Oneness we are "God", who also can imagine itself as one god among many. The power of the imagination is inexhaustible. Living in this absolute reality as God, as oneness, we can create new relative realities, then enter into them and imagine that we have forgotten that we are actually God and live in oneness.

What an exciting game! We can enter into the imaginations created by all of us – thus also created by me myself as an individual – or we can create brand-new imaginations, just as we please. All choices are open to us. We can also create conscious souls that see themselves in very different bodies. We are able to create anything that we are able to imagine.

When we now ask those being in the trance state to tell why we have somehow removed ourselves from this All-Oneness, we get the following explanation: While living in this unity, in which we experience total blissfulness, total peace, total love and total harmony, we can only enjoy these qualities if we also experience the opposite, namely suffering, conflict, lovelessness, disharmony, as well as all the variations developing from these constellations. Therefore, in order to always experience this totality of all-harmony and all-love, we create in our playful mood entities in which we recognize ourselves as beings separated from one another and therefore standing in contrast to that divine unity.[38]

This is the real reason for all human experience on earth. With our divine power we have created ourselves. In order to feel the desolation of the soul, the loneliness immanent in the suffering while experiencing separation from unity, we have created at the same time forgetfulness of our real origin. Nevertheless we maintain in our separation an inkling of that realization, namely that a higher state still exists with which we are still somehow connected. Thus the longing to

38. Another very original ontological standpoint is offered by the teacher and reincarnation therapist Professor Kurt Tepperwein. When we are in unity, and thus totally in accordance with the divine, everything we do is always in harmony with the One. Then everything that we can think and do always fits into the divine plan. Here there is no more freedom of choice, for we know what is right and behave accordingly. But - out of the playful mood of again freely choosing between what is in accordance with the divine plan and what is not – we begin from the beginning - a "repeat performance" which could be called "finding through free will my way back to God's will". – A further ontological-spiritual approach may be found in Aurobindo`s *Der integrale Yoga.* (p. 52 ff.)

be reunited with the higher state is still latent in our being.

We can experience this opposite of the divine all-harmony and all-love in the most different dimensions, according to the structures of space and time created by our imagination. And we can experience ourselves simultaneously even in different dimensions and forms, depending on how highly our imaginative powers are activated. Together with all others, we can also create a higher mental supervisor as our Higher Self, which again cares for the many bodies containing souls.

Many dimensions have already been imagined by us, i.e. by the unity, so that these already created spaces and times can be reoccupied and filled with new creations. And we have already entered our imagined worlds many times or an unlimited number of times, for in the unity everyone is everyone else and all are one. Thus every imagination is also my imagination. In unity I am in my divinity everything, and all my imaginations are our imaginations, and all the other imaginations are simultaneously my imaginations. There is no separation – unless it is an imagined separation.

To be able to experience the different imagined dimensions we need a form or a body. But to experience in our bodies and to store and accumulate the experiences we need a soul. In contrast to the eternal being as the spiritual principle the soul is the constantly growing principle, while matter, including the earthly body, is the constantly changing principle.

Establishment of rules for the play of karma

The plan created for experiencing the opposite of ourselves may be briefly outlined as follows:

1. **Living in the All-Oneness.** Decision to experience the opposite of divine all-harmony and all-love. Voluntary choice for the law of karma. **Fundamental Karma.**
2. **Life as a stone, plant or animal.** Slumbering consciousness. **Karma-free existence.** No freedom of will, but experience of the opposite of divine all-harmony and all-love. As an animal guided by instincts. As a mammal already beginning of training for free choice.
3. **Life as a human.** Subject to the law of cause and effect. **Life-karma.** Production of karma by voluntary violation of the law of love; thus self-caused karmic reaction. Conditioning to proper action through experience. Through karmic reaction experience of the opposite of divine all-harmony and all-love.
4. **Life in the beyond.** Convalescence, feedback, preparation for new incarnation. Free or partially free choice of type and distribution of karmic events in coming life. **Karma planning.**

In the state of unity and All-Oneness, in the all-mental existence, we have established a complete plan for the contrast program we would like to experience, including the karmic events we plan to experience as a human being. Thus our fundamental karma is already set here.

Thus everyone has already conceived his own plan in the mental dimension before incarnating. (Plotinus prefers to see this act of plan-conceiving in the Nous, i.e. the mental foundation of the imagination.) So the "rules of the game" are set up – and in the coming game we will follow these rules. As soon as we have decided to carry out the game to the end, there will be no way out, just as there is no exit from a flying airplane. At the end of the game everyone will be the winner, no matter how long he or she has played. One player may be finished before another – even if they started at the same time. Others we overtake on the way may have already been active before we began.

Upon reaching the goal, we will reawaken consciously in the All-Oneness. All of our imagined separation as well as our longing for unity will be over. Our return is equivalent to reawakening in the divine All-Oneness. By means of this game of karma we will have experienced the opposite of all-harmony and all-love and are able again fully to enjoy our state as part (or better as no-part) of the "All-Divine".

Experience of the opposite of the divine all-harmony before our first incarnation as human

If we enter into a dimension such as that in which e.g. the earth is found, we can choose whether to take a longer or a shorter path, depending on how much or how quickly we would like to experience the opposite of the divine all-harmony.

And in each appearance in such a form we experience a beginning, a birth, as well as an end, a death. These also belong to the opposite of the divine unity – in which there is no time, no beginning, no transition and therefore also no death. Because we want to experience the opposite of all-harmony and all-love for the benefit of the whole, we can decide to begin, e.g. on the planet earth, from the very beginning, connecting our imagination with material elements – such as water or earth or stones. As such we can feel the attraction of the earth's gravity, thus feeling captured and immobile. Since time has no meaning for us, a few million years would make no difference. So we learn patience.

And then, if we have so planned, we can also enter into all different kinds of plants, whose forms are already given to us at the time we are in the All-Oneness. Here, too, we experience the opposite of the divine all-harmony, being subject to the changing weather as well as to sprouting, growing and withering away. We can expand ourselves but are still bound to a certain plot of land.

After that we can, if we have chosen, enter into so-to-speak "prefabricated" animal forms in order to also experience a lot about the opposite of unity: e.g. the fear of being killed by another animal or by man, the fear of not getting enough to eat, in general the fear of not maintaining our body – and naturally the greatest fear of all, fear of death. I believe that we already experience as an animal the greatest external fears as the opposite of all-harmony and all-love.

As rocks and minerals, plants and animals we still have no individual consciousness and can thus cause no karmic reactions, but we still experience most of the aspects of the opposition to all-harmony and all-love.

This doesn't mean that these experiences of the soul are only effected by the opposite of all-harmony and all-love. Because we also experience in these bodies much beauty and much love, e.g. the pleasure and joy of the plant at sunrise, the joys of motherhood or the exuberance of young animals. But this happiness can also be suddenly taken away. The danger of a changing situation is always present, possibly bringing about suffering.

We only give a brief summary here, as the complete details would exceed the scope of the present investigation. It may suffice to say that plants and animals serve to extend the experience of the contrast to all-harmony and all-love for all beings. And they themselves also profit from this experience. They have a total-soul, a species-soul and can have an individual soul, if they are also implanted with a soul that wants to develop later into a human – which not every plant-soul or animal-soul will do. But house pets are generally souls prepared for becoming humans.

And not every human must have been a stone, plant or animal before becoming a human for the first time. One can also voluntarily decide from the start to incarnate as a human, entering the "karma game" at this high level at one's own risk and without extensive preparation in other life forms.

In the first part of this book we already discussed the great extent to which Indian thought has occupied itself with reincarnation in animal or plant bodies. This experience of the transition through the plant and animal form before attaining a human body is not only described in the ancient Vedas but has been taught by later authorities from the founder of Sufism, Dschaladin Rumi, on down to Sai Baba.

And Regression Research confirms this, for many of those treated by me (also in the group seminars) have experienced themselves as stones, plants and/or animals – even in multiple lives. But I have to reject the belief that we are demoted again to the plant or animal level because of misdeeds. These beliefs have not been confirmed in Regression Therapy and should be buried in the graveyard of mythology.

Subjection to the karmic law of cause and effect as a human

It is possible to experience the opposite of all-harmony only in the plant or animal form. But if it is part of our plan, we will sooner or later incarnate as a human. In the human form we experience a number of opposites to divine harmony and love, e.g. jealousy, greed, hate, envy, despair, lovesickness, fear of punishment, fear of not being accepted or loved by others, loneliness, hopelessness (a type of mental derangement) and many other things causing suffering, fear and psychic pains. Even the a woman's labor pains at the birth of a new child belong to the experience of the opposite of divine harmony.

We experience, of course, not only the opposite of the divine all-harmony and all-love. Because in every life there are also positive experiences and feelings to encourage us and keep us going in the ups and downs we have to live through here. But even the most wonderful feelings and experiences offer only a poor picture of what the divine all-harmony and all-love really have in store for us. Subconsciously we know about them, and a steadily growing premonition from life to life keeps alive our desire to experience them.

Finally the individual attains its first human form as pre-established in the preceding period of the beyond. This is perhaps the first of many such forms we will need to finally reach our goal. But on our long journey there are also other consolations: Every day is interrupted by night, a period of relaxation during which we can recuperate in sleep for the challenges of the coming day, challenges in which we repeatedly experience the opposite of the divine all-harmony and all-love. And as the days are interrupted by nights, also different earthly lives are interrupted by a pause, an intermediate period in the beyond, created by us all in the All-Oneness, in which we can recuperate before entering a new life full of facets of the opposite of the divine unity.

But this experience of the opposite would only be a mechanical and monotonous game if there were no development, no end, and no aim.

We have subjected ourselves to certain special rules for this period as a human being. And we do not want the total experience of the opposite of the total harmony in just one lifetime. This would be too much for us and would not even be possible. So we divide it into several or many lifetimes, recuperating between times in the beyond. Our experience of the opposite of all-harmony and all-love is, however, always dependent on one condition: We must always act in free will, at least as much as possible. And although we always strive to experience more of the opposite of harmony, we want to decide ourselves in which steps we would like to do it.

It was our ingenious preplanned[39] idea of allowing ourselves also to experience from life to life on earth more and more of the divine love already presented to us in the unity. And the more we let go of our ego-centeredness, the more we remember of our experience of all-love in the All-Oneness.

Whenever we act in a callous way against the love speaking to us through our inner voice or feeling, we ourselves will have to experience exactly the same punishment directed against us. The law of karma will be brought into play, teaching us what it means to be treated in a loveless way. And at the same time our need to experience

---

39. Plotinus speaks of the Nous, a universal consciousness emanating from the One to produce the world of Ideas, which latter then becomes equipped with the world soul and individual souls. This may actually be correct. Further investigations in reincarnation therapy will show if Plotinus also found the truth in this case.

the opposite of divine all-harmony and all-love is fulfilled. This is a perfect combination of our overriding will and previous decision to serve the Whole through experience of the opposite of the Divine Love, on the one hand, and, on the other, our own personal free will as human beings: to decide to do what our inner love actually demands of us in accordance with the Divine Will, i.e. our own higher will.

In order to learn as much as possible from the opposite, we have fitted ourselves out with a strong ego desiring to fulfill self-centered earthly needs and wishes – even in opposition to the needs of others. We already learned to have this ego – which repeatedly commits offenses against love – during our (probable) time as an animal. We have chosen such an ego because through such loveless deeds we cause ourselves to have the experiences in balancing lives as a victim that we actually out of our own higher decision want to have. Thus the acts that we carry out as perpetrators are based on our own higher will. We are not actually at fault in carrying out callous deeds. No, we are still in agreement with our original decision to entangle ourselves in the karmic law – in order to register the necessary painful experiences in our soul.

And as we heard in Case 2, we have to experience as humans all different aspects in the cycle of our repeated earthly lives in order to make a "polished diamond" of ourselves. These experiences of the soul are what are necessary to bring us back to divine unity, instilling the knowledge of its opposite in the divine unity itself.

Beginning in ignorance, we set out on the adventurous journey, making our first steps. These will be followed by many incarnations. Our intention is by exercising our freedom of will to learn gradually to walk the divine way of love. Every other path will lead us to suffering, but will also allow us to experience the opposite of the divine unity. So the law of karma gradually conditions us to do good, allowing us to exercise our own freedom of will. Thereby we experience, on the one hand, that everything done against love will make us suffer and, on the other hand, that we will profit from everything we do on earth out of love and in agreement with the divine laws.

Thus everything rests on our free decision, whether we experience suffering or joy. And after many earthly lives of having gone through the different painful paths of conditioning, we will have finally learned to listen to our inner voice. We are now looking for the way out of this wheel of reincarnation (*and if the reader would not be right now on such a path, he/she would hardly have picked up a book like the present one*).

And the way out of the cycle of birth and rebirth is very simple: LOVE. This is the magic word. Everyone who has completely grasped the basis of this game – i.e. from ego-consciousness to us-consciousness, from lovelessness to love – will reach the same insight. And Regression Therapy sessions allow such insights from a higher level, because we can suddenly become part of this higher consciousness on the Mountain of Revelation.

I would like to summarize the karmic process once more by an example:

The karmic dance on the rope of love

There is a tightrope hanging over a deep abyss over which the karma-dancer has to walk. The side from which he begins to walk with his balancing rod is the side of ignorance, of ego-centeredness, of lack of love. The balancing rod is his conscience. If he knows how to use it properly, it will help him to avoid stumbling. On the other side of the abyss wait wisdom, universal consciousness, all-love, unity. And now he begins his balancing act on this tightrope of karma. If he can retain a loving attitude, he will be able to cross the rope quickly to the other side. But as soon as he commits an offense against love in thought or word, there will be some greater or smaller degree of shakiness, which he may be able to balance out with help of the balancing rod. But as soon as he acts against love, he will fall from the rope to the left or right side. The greater his offense, the deeper he falls. But karmic providence may also lift him with the same force back onto the rope – this is karmic resolution.

And when he returns to the rope, he can continue walking. Subconsciously he knows what has caused his fall, so he will now be careful not to repeat the same mistake. Every step that he takes while carrying out loving thoughts and deeds will make him advance a little on the rope. And every major act of love moves him a good bit further. But at one time or another he will forget his caution, causing him to fall again. He will have to feel again and again the re-establishing power in the form of karma, setting him again back onto the rope. Because no one can really fall into eternal damnation – we are protected from that by the divine love.

So gradually he balances on and on across the rope, sometimes falling off to the right or left, but again and again being returned by the balancing law of karma. He knows that he will have to reach the other side eventually. Because there is no turning back.

Arriving in the middle of the rope, he can take several

steps forward without falling, though he may occasionally waver. But now he doesn't begin to sway or fall off so often – the more his love develops, the surer of himself he becomes on the rope, making fewer and fewer offenses against love. He learns more and more to trust his balancing rod, making up quickly for any vacillations. Gradually he becomes a master of the tightrope, dancing with pleasure there and finally even throwing his rod away while balancing with his out-streched arms. But the longing to reach the complete state of love on the other side – overriding even his joy in dancing – is now so great in him that with brisk, sure steps he takes the last few steps to the goal drawn like a magnet by a higher source of love at the other end. And arms of love are reaching for him there, awaiting him with joy, hugging him and praising him. Because he has reached his goal, sinking into the embraces of universal love. He has returned home, back to Godhead, the total All-Oneness.

The meaning of love for the karmic law

As we have just demonstrated in this little parable of the rope of karma (an Indian would rather speak of the rope of *dharma* [religious practice of the right path]), the law of karma helps us to learn not to leave the path of love but to stay on it. It aims to remind us not to make the same mistakes again and again.

Thus karma is only a means to an end, namely to lead us on the basis of our preceding free choices first to the experience of the opposite of the divine unity and finally to the proper decisions and actions in accordance with the divine laws of harmony and love. Karma is therefore no principle of punishment but one of education, or even better: a support-system for returning us to true love. The

Bhagavad-Gita says already [40]:

> But beyond this life there is another, eternal, invisible,
> Which, though all beings are destroyed, is never destroyed.
> Invisible, eternal, it is also called the final goal.
> When reached, one never returns: Look, this is My supreme abode!
> The Supreme Spirit is attained by love alone for Him
> Who created all and in Whom all we are.

We must distinguish, as mentioned above, between three types of acceptance of karma:

- our acceptance of karma in the original unity, allowing us to experience disharmony and lack of love and leading to our original karmic burden;
- our acceptance on the earthly level, where our consciousness is unaware of our real destination and the meaning of our presence on earth, but where we also always have the possibility to choose between the proper – i.e. loving – and the improper – i.e. ego-centered and loveless – attitude; and finally
- our acceptance in each period of the beyond between lives on earth concerning that which is to be experienced in the individual coming earth life (cf. details below).

The game of life is thus based on free decisions made on all of these three levels. Everything has a meaning, for there is nothing in God's creation that is meaningless. Even if we humans carry out so-called "senseless" actions, they do have the result that we recognize later – if only in the

40. Bhagavadgita, Song 8, Couplets 20 –22.

beyond – their senselessness. We learn from our mistakes, for which reason we should never curse them but rather seek to avoid them in the future. The same is true of wrong actions leading to karmic reactions. Because the law "What you have done to others, you have done to yourself" still remains valid – in respect to positive as well as negative actions.

The law of karma was not created by us in the original state of unity in order to punish ourselves. Its purpose was tő sharpen our awareness and our senses in respect to our actions. If we remove ourselves from love, we will be removed from it, too. If we open ourselves to love, we will be given more love. Karma of the negative is nothing else but actions that were carried out without love and that have not yet been balanced by love. By loveless actions we can learn the value of love.

Ulli (Case 11) made this realization during the Regression Therapy session when he heard that as a result of his callous life as Fopar his soul had had to experience in his victim's life as the prostitute what it was like to be unloved and therefore stoned to death. In this way the soul's desire for love is increased.

Life as a school of karma

We could compare every life of a soul with a day in school – the "school of karma". The major subject studied there every day is love. Of course there are also other minor subjects, such as patience, moderation, creativity, tolerance etc. In this school we learn through ever-new interactions and role-plays better and better how to keep our ego under control and more and more to open ourselves to love. The many written exams that we have to turn into the teacher have corrected and handed back. The mistakes he marks are those against love. Later on we have the chance to repeat these tasks until we are able to pass the tests without a mistake.

The teacher doesn't scold us for our mistakes, no matter how bad they are, but rather he points them out to us kindly and lovingly. But there is no way around the need to learn how to avoid these mistakes. And when one part of the curriculum has been mastered, the next one is waiting. If we are lazy, perhaps we will fail and have to repeat, perhaps even several times. But no one is sent back to a lower level. Because what we have once learned, we cannot forget. How much we learn at any one time only depends on our free decision. But at the end everyone will graduate. Not everyone will receive a report card with the highest marks, but everyone will have attained the goal. In more advanced schools or universities (in the beyond) we will perfect our knowledge further. And sooner or later we will become masters in that which we have studied, namely Masters of Love.[41]

Of the effects of karma in everyday life

The great Greek thinker Pythagoras was initiated into esoteric secrets in Egypt, probably also learning there to recall his earlier lives. He not only gave us the well-known laws of acoustic harmony and the mathematical formula $a^2+b^2=c^2$ but understood also the law of karma already 500 years before Christ – apparently even before its appearance

41. Sai Baba also likes to use the example of school in connection with karma, „So-called negative karma is like school grades which show how much you know or how much you have been able to put into practice" (v. Stepski-Doliwa IV, p. 260).

in India (!) – because he says, "The result of all good deeds of a person squared plus the result of the result of all bad deeds squared equals the total of the square opposite to the right angle in a following life."[42]

What a fitting answer! Here there is nothing of the punishment or reprisal later present in the Indian karma concept. It is nothing more or less than the statement that the good and bad results are summed up and take effect in a following life according to the good and bad actions in the former life.

---

42. Unfortunately I am no longer able to find the source for this quote. Even if it was only approximately said in this way, it would have great consequences for karma research. We know that he was able to remember exactly his earlier lives (e.g. participation in the Trojan War). We also know that he received his knowledge as an initiate in an Egyptian temple (Sais?). After returning to Greece, he became the first Greek philosopher to teach reincarnation (even before Socrates). He founded his own mystery cult, in which he distinguished between those disciples of his only to receive general esoteric knowledge – the "Exoterics" – and those to receive special knowledge under oath of secrecy – the "Esoterics".
It seems probable that at that time the concept of reincarnation already existed in India but was still lacking the karmic components which were not obvious until the appearance of the Mahabharata and of Buddhism and Jainism – i.e. probably not earlier than the 4th century, B.C. – but which then gradually began to influence Indian thought more and more.
Egypt already had had economic connections with India for many centuries. Is it possible that Egyptian secret priest schools had other disciples like Pythagoras also from India who received the idea of karma with their initiation, later mixing it with their own concept of Indian reincarnation? Is it thus possible that not India but Egypt is the birthplace of the idea of karma? Did not Herodotus refer to the fact that the idea of reincarnation stems from Egypt? Scientists should delve into these questions to find out if these suppositions can be substantiated or not.

Is this statement of Pythagoras still true in light of the facts uncovered in Regression Therapy? The answer is: "Yes" – and "No". Everything bad or good that we humans cause on the basis of our free decision has an effect on our karma. For instance, if I help a blind woman in crossing a dangerous street, I will receive at some time in this or in a following life a similar service. If I steal something, something will have to be stolen from me. Our good and bad deeds are kept in an invisible karma account-book[43] of the soul. On the one side there are our credits, on the other our debits, or in Pythagoras' terms: a^2 and b^2. And, as we will see later in connection with preparations in the beyond for a coming life on earth, some parts will be taken from the credit side of our account and some from the debit side, so that a combination is evolved fitting to the life in question. But at some time the debit side will have to be eliminated. This is part of the rules already established in the All-Oneness.

Whatever has been balanced out on the debit side is erased, the soul no longer being held accountable for it. But the sum on the credit side is accumulated – plus interest.

Thus the account for the following life is not $a^2+b^2=c^2$, but c^2 is variable, varying according to the amount I would like to learn - under consideration of what a^2 and b^2 have already amounted to in the previous life. And I would also like to add a comment from Sai Bàba to this: "If you have not saved anything, if nothing has been deposited to your 'karma-account', there will be nothing there for an

43. Rudolf Steiner speaks of the fact that, if possible, one should already strive on earth to „get some good marks entered into one's book of life". (Hummel, p. 92)

emergency. So begin today to deposit something to your account. Speak the truth. Be upright."[44]

The law of karma is the spiritual law of cause and effect, having exactly the same effect as the physical law of cause and effect formulated by Isaac Newton. The higher the place from which a stone falls, the deeper the hole it will make on falling. And the worse you act towards love, the worse are the reactions you will have to suffer. It's that simple.

The law of karma is not to be understood as punishment, just as the law of gravity is no punishment. It is simply a law, therefore without bias. Of course one can speak of the "relentless" law of karma, as the Cyprian mystic Daskalos does: "All incarnations with which I have had to do show me that the law is relentlessly at work."[45] But who would like to call the law of gravity "relentless"? Surely no one. It is simply a law. And we should accept the law of karma in the same way. Because now we know from where it comes and for what reason it has come into being.

The whole of the original knowledge about our source and our destination is anchored in our subconscious. But for wise reasons it has been covered over for many lives by our ego. The more we reduce our ego, the more of our original knowledge comes to light.

Writing a karmic check on our account always means an offense against love. If we are able to equalize it by love in time, it may – depending on the circumstances – be possible to lighten the karmic load or eliminate it again. There are also other possibilities to correct our karma, which however

44. v. Stepski-Doliwa IV, p. 62
45. Markides I, p. 155f

require an advanced state of consciousness. Under normal circumstances, for instance, it is not possible to accept the karmic load of another person. This is only possible – under certain conditions – for the very advanced. So once Daskalos accepted the karmic illness of his grandson. And Kirpal Singh is said to have accepted the sanchit-karma, i.e. the karma carried subconsciously into a future life, of his disciples so that they could make faster spiritual progress. But both Daskalos and Kirpal Singh had to experience their reactions, causing for the former a short illness but for the latter long-term suffering.[46]

Under normal circumstances no one can avoid the consequences of an action, for the reaction will come sooner or later. The law of karma is more exacting than earthly justice. We are the sowers. As we prepare the field and sow the seeds, so we will reap the harvest. "Everyone must eat the fruits of his own field."[47] And every seed sprouts. If I sow poison ivy, I cannot expect to get daisies as my harvest. Even if I plant an apple tree, still I cannot expect to pluck mangoes from the branches. Therefore I have to be careful at planting time what I would like to reap, for the harvest is mine alone. So I cannot sell or give the fruits away if they do not taste good to me. I have to eat the harvest all by myself.

The law of karma is just as neutral as electricity. It only depends on me how I would like to use it. I can use it as light to drive away the darkness or even to illuminate a festival that I have graciously prepared out of love for others. Or I can use the current for electro-shocks to

---

46. Darshan Singh,
47. Liz Green in Hanson, p. 163

torture others with. I have my own free will to manage the current as I like. But whatever I do to others will also be done to me, though I may have to wait a few lives for it.

We learn to use electric current by comparing the experiences we have with it. The same is true of the karma law. But it is of no use to be told by others what to do or not to do. What others say may be right or wrong – we can only learn by our own experience.

The effect that an electric shock has on different persons also varies greatly. One person may receive "the shock of his lifetime", whereas another may remain unfazed. The same is true of the law of karma. Military service, for instance, may be a great pleasure for one, but for another it may be hell. In a prisoner-of-war camp one may afterwards be grateful for having grown in experiences, while someone else considers that his life is ruined for the rest of his days. And for karmic reasons we will always react to situations in the way the karmic reaction requires. If as a prison guard in an earlier life I tortured others, I will have to suffer from my time as a prisoner in a later life just as much as the persons I mistreated earlier.

Because the law of karma has us to experience just the same results as we have caused, we are met by just the same things that we have applied to others. For this reason it is known often as retributive – a term that Indian authors as well as Helena P. Blavatsky have used[48]. The word retribution has a repressive note. In agreement with Dick Sutphen I prefer the term "balancing". Because it is not a question of punishment for callous deeds, but of a counteracting of mistaken actions, whether they were

48. Diana Dunningham Chapotin in Hanson, p. 183

intentional or not.

Intentional mistaken actions in the form of "boomerang karma" (as Edgar Cayce calls it), in which that which I do returns to me, are naturally worse than unintentional ones. Intentional actions in contradiction to one's inner voice make the action worse. But for the process of learning it is also important to be confronted with one's unintentional mistakes, in order to learn how one should actually act in such a situation.

The law of karma is "the law according to which we have to accept the inheritance of our own past".[49] We inherit from life to life what we have done before. Whoever therefore would like to have a good inheritance, should organize his life so that what he leaves behind is positive. The law of karma is, as we saw in connection with the analogy of "walking the tight-rope", a law that re-establishes a balance. Every imbalance in the universe has to be brought back into harmonious balance. In the same way every misdeed of a person must be re-balanced. The harmony disturbed in a life as a perpetrator must be re-established in a life as a victim. Only when I am able to live perfectly in accordance with the divine law of harmony and love do I no longer get out of balance and need "re-balancing". Then I act in accordance with the divine laws in me.

Just as the law of karma is neutral, it is also unbiased toward everyone. Because it is incorruptible, being justice itself. Everyone receives exactly what he deserves – on the basis of his own earlier, free decision. And nothing happens to anyone in life that he does not deserve. Even if someone

49. Virginia Hanson in Hanson, p. 254

who is not guilty is condemned by a court, under karmic considerations the decision is completely just. This may be called cosmic justice, because it is based on a higher jurisdiction. And we have already mentioned of the way in which this law is derived. Because we ourselves have created it at our original source, or at least agreed to it because we wanted to experience the opposite of all-harmony and all-love.

Now we can understand why Angelica (Case 2) could say from higher insight that it was not a question of justice but of existence itself. Because in our lives as a perpetrator we experience through our misdeeds the fact of our misuse of power and love. We actually even needed to load ourselves with negative karma. We required this experience in order to encounter in the balancing lives as a victim our own negative acts – the opposite of the divine harmony and love – turned against us ourselves. And we also need the respective balance in our life as a victim in order to develop our own desire to strive for love, after experiencing the lack of love in actions turned against us. Because that which we lack is what we most earnestly desire.

The advantages of the law of karma

"Karma is a wonder in its precision with the intention in making you think and thus follow the right path."[50] It offers us practical training through examples. It applies pressure to make us see what we lack. And what we lack is...more love! There is no punishment, only correction. The law of karma offers us the chance to expand our knowledge and love. It speeds our development; indeed

50. v.Stepski-Doliwa IV, p. 332

without this law we would not be able to develop. We would just keep on eternally allowing our ego to carry out its malicious games, with only the earthly laws to restrict it.

The law of karma blames no one. The blame lies only in being not yet a good student who, makes many mistakes. And these mistakes are only reversible through time itself. I cannot blame anyone else, be it God, fate or individual situations. Because I myself was the agent – without guilt because I was still ignorant, immature or too weak to control my ego and its malicious games. Perpetrators are often to be considered like irresponsible children. Spiritually immature, they rarely develop pangs of conscience for their acts until shortly before or often only after death. A bad conscience is essential to motivate them to experience the same acts done against themselves. And only then can there be balancing.

Angelica's soul (Case 2) experienced, for instance, after its life as a Russian merchant and callous egomaniac great remorse. And at the same time it was suddenly moved by the love surrounding it. And it knew that all feelings of guilt melt away under the influence of love: "Love heals all wounds."

Karma is the horizontal principle, for it remains on the earth. Dharma is the way of righteousness, the moral source leading us upward to the divine, to higher realms of love. Annie Besant, the director of the world Theosophical Society, once said that karma pushes us from the past while dharma pulls us on to the future.[51]

51. Quote by William Metzger in Hanson, p. 194. The same author also uses dharma as a vertical and karma as a horizontal axis (p. 195).

The law of karma is meant to teach us responsibility. Every day we must decide what is right and what is wrong. We have to learn to listen to our own inner wisdom, to the inner voice telling us as our conscience how we should act. This inner voice often doesn't fit our present attitude - or is even bothersome – and many try to divert themselves from it, if necessary with the help of alcohol etc.

Many of us are used to accepting in agreement with our egoistic desires authorities from without. In the Middle Ages we were glad, for instance, to accept the call of the Church: "Burn the witches, the Jews, the heretics." We were angry at someone or something and took the call of worldly authorities as a welcome occasion to release our aggressions. And we willingly ignored the inner voice telling us not to take part in such excesses, using as an excuse that it was the Church as God's representative that had initiated them.

And what authorities do we use today as our excuses when we are driven by ego to break the laws of love? The church, politicians, press, our parents or even the ancient Holy Scriptures? Actually we can only claim our own conscience as our authority. The law of karma teaches us out of experience to be purely concerned with loving others, to take responsibility for all our thoughts, words and actions.

On my way through my many earthly lives I am responsible for my own progress. I may determine myself how fast I would like to reach my goal. I carry the full responsibility and am the master of my own fortune. And the law of karma helps me to learn faster what are the really important things. So now we can understand why Sai Baba can say, "Consider always that everything that occurs to you is also the best for you. Your task is to find out why."[52]

But first we want to find out what types of karma actually exist.

The 23 Types of Karma

For every karmic event there must be a previous cause, which then manifests itself as a karmic effect. There are twenty-three different types of karmic events, as listed in the following pages:

1. **The Original karma** (Ur-Karma) is, as extensively described above, chosen by us before our taking a human body – or actually even before leaving the original unity. We desired to become aware of what the One offered as all-harmony and all-love by experiencing its opposite. This experience of the opposite of divine harmony and love are important, so that we can enjoy these further. We do not wish, however, to live through this opposite in just one "go", and we also wish to combine this experience with our free will. Sai Baba hits the nail on the head when he says, "The free will of man requires him to not learn by precept but only by means of that which he experiences and lives through. ...Reincarnation and karma exist so that everyone has the chance to learn from his own mistakes."[53]

   Everything that happens in life serves a higher as well as an earthly purpose. As souls we have joined the game of incarnation – whose rules are determined by

52. v. Stepski-Doliwa, III, p. 101
53. v. Stepski-Doliwa IV, p. 225

the law of karma – with the intention of experiencing not only the pleasant, but also the unpleasant sides of the game. The purpose of the law of karma is to lead us from hard-heartedness on to love, but we have to find the way ourselves! Because everything is One, the soul of man – as part of this One – has planned this all himself out of his own free will.

So if one is in a balancing life as a victim, this can be composed of many different lives as a perpetrator, which may be carried out in different ways, as follows: In one life a) the full balancing of a life as a perpetrator can take place; b) several acts of hard-heartedness from different lives can be made up for completely; c) only a part of the life as a perpetrator to be balanced can appear; d) several different parts of different lives as a perpetrator can be balanced; e) a mixture of all these can take place at once; f) different balancing events from lives as a perpetrator can manifest themselves along with (different) repercussions from lives as a victim (cf. above: Cases 3, 13 and 26).

2. **Balancing karma** is what is generally known under the name "karma", namely: "What you have done to another, you have (actually) done to yourself"; "As ye sow, so shall ye reap". Thus one may speak of "boomerang karma" (Edgar Cayce) or "retaliation karma" (Blavatsky). Indians like to call it "praraghda-karma".

Balancing karma follows the law of cause and effect, and one receives reactions himself in accordance with one's negative and positive actions towards others. The cases described in Part 3 are primarily concerned with this kind of karma. But we have been mainly concerned with the negative side of karma because in most cases the clients were driven to seek therapy by the negative reactions in their lives as victims, which of course were only the result of their lives as perpetrators.

Perpetrators and victims are dependent on each other: the perpetrator needs a victim in order to sin against love; the victim needs a perpetrator in order to rid himself of his karmic burden. So one generally experiences in therapy a previous life as a perpetrator, in which one maliciously raped, killed, committed arson or fraud, lied etc. This life is naturally followed by a life of (negative) karmic reactions. But it is only very seldom true that – as Kabir thought – the perpetrator by injuring the victim causes the victim to return himself as a perpetrator who then returns the same injury to his former perpetrator.

As demonstrated by many of the cases shown here, the perpetrator may often be a rapist, returning in one of his next lives as a woman, who is then raped herself. Here it could be asked which of the two we should pity more: the woman who has just been raped and who will suffer greatly from this but who has now been able to rid herself of her karmic burden? Or perhaps the new perpetrator, who has just taken upon himself a karmic burden and must now reincarnate one or more times as a woman in order to experience being raped? The latter still has his karmic reaction in front of him. And such a reaction is inevitable.

The law of karma knows no exceptions. As we have

seen, it is generally men who take upon themselves karmic guilt. And in most cases (as also in those shown here) these souls are women when they have to experience their experience of karmic balancing..

3. **Karmic after-effects:** This kind of karma applies to positive as well as to negative side effects. But in this context we mean primarily by this term all those additional effects – and mainly the negative ones - that stem from a life of a victim and are still activating themselves in the same or more often in a following life as karmic after-effects.

   If, for example, a woman in an life as a victim is supposed to have as a karmic reaction the experience of being raped, then there can be various other accompanying circumstances that will themselves again have repercussions later on. If the rape of a girl collecting berries in the forest is carried out by three men (Case 13), there may be after-effects in her next life such as the fear of walking alone in a forest, distaste for berries or fear of meeting three men while alone. And sexual complexes or hate of all men may remain, causing her to stay unmarried. Perhaps she will also avoid wearing make-up to keep men from taking notice of her.

   Or another example: Robbers attack a man in his carriage. He is pulled out and knifed from behind into the heart. If reborn as a man, he may have heart problems today as a direct result of this death. But in an earlier life he himself may have thrust his sword into someone else's heart. Thus his experience in the life as a victim was a major balancing event, while his present heart problems are to be seen as a balancing after-effect of the life as a victim, belonging still to the balancing karmic reactions, but as a subsequent part event. The experience of that death impressed itself as further after-effects in his emotional body: not only does he possibly have a birthmark of the size of the point of the knife at the place where it entered his back, but he has also developed a fear of knives and an iron-allergy. In addition, he has the habit of always standing or sitting with his back to the wall or otherwise protected from attack from behind. When he is outside, he turns involuntarily every minute or two to make sure no one is slipping up on him. These additional signs of the karmic balancing event, such as (compulsive) habits, allergies, fears and phobias, belong to the karmic after-effects.

Those he had attacked as a perpetrator could, of course, also have acquired all these behavior patterns and mannerisms. Thus they would also already be anchored in his life as a perpetrator. At any rate, most karmic after-effects obviously have their own individual meaning, which may also be connected with other, earlier lives and must be considered in the context of the whole.

Another case from Part 3 of the present book: Angelica (Case 2) had raped young girls in her life as a Russian maritime merchant. In lives as a (female) victim she was raped herself several times. Though her present hay fever is a result of these rapes, it is an after-effect of the life as a victim and only indirectly connected to the life as a perpetrator. Most of the clients who come to Regression Therapy are burdened

– and quite often heavily – by karmic after-effects from their lives as a victim.

Such after-effects of karmic balancing events can be of different types: a) body marks (stigmata), i.e. birth defects without laming (laming would probably imply "balancing karma"); b) psychic symptoms, e.g. bad dreams and compulsive habits; c) emotional symptoms, e. g. most fears and inexplicable emotional reactions; d) unusual behavior patterns, e.g. rejection of a certain country because of a cruel death there, without being consciously aware of it today.

But of course these karmic after-effects include not only negative things, actions and people, but also the after-effects of positive earlier experiences, comprising among other things inexplicable preferences and attractions - usually without negative tinges. Often we may think these after-effects to be inherited, but in my opinion they are self-germinating seeds from earlier lives. For instance we could have developed a talent for music or handicrafts by having occupied ourselves with it for many lives. Or a love of animals could stem from many lives in which we were associated with animals and learned to appreciate them.

"Inborn" talents such as riding, sailing, swimming etc. also derive from already acquired abilities. Usually one's life is made up of numerous positive and negative karmic after-effects, so that one may "jump for joy" one day and be "down in the dumps" the next. Our life is made up of myriad positive and negative effects from earlier lives, which sum up to a kaleidoscope of multi-colored pebbles with a few black ones thrown in for good measure. We are the sum of all our previous experiences, and they can all pop up again – anytime – when the right trigger appears.

Everything that exists is made up of vibrations. When the vibrations of positive or negative events from an earlier life become registered and stored in the emotional body, they can be reactivated if: a) the same vibration turns up again (e.g. sudden panic when one's child approaches a "dangerous" slope), b) there is similarity (e.g. rejection of a person who looks like or awakens the same feelings as someone already subconsciously registered as being unpleasant), c) there is a vibrational association awakening a previously dormant karmic reaction.

Perhaps the reader will remember the milk as the carrier of vibrations reawakening a negative reaction of the hemorrhoids (Case 24). Or when Ulli (Case 11) suddenly panicked from the vibrations of the stones combined with the effect of closeness and darkness. Similar vibrations in his emotional body suddenly resonated setting the karmic process into action again and reawakening his tendency to panic.

All Indian "samskaras" must also be counted among these after-effect reactions: impressions such as "scars and idiosyncrasies", which have been "created, maintained and formed", as the Indologist Heinrich Zimmer would say. Everything that I possess as personal traits or preferences, also my fears, interests and abilities must have been created at some point in time. Normally they stem from earlier lives or – as we will see later – from things learned in the "beyond".

4. **Sacrificial karma** is karma unrelated to one's own person. That is, a soul can offer to aid some other soul who is reincarnating by teaching it or helping it to learn something. A concrete example: Perhaps unloving parents of a child let it starve in an earlier life or let it be neglected or abandoned, so that it suffered terribly. In the beyond those parents will realize how unloving they were towards their child. In them there will be coming up a longing to make up for their neglect by wanting a child in their next life to whom they would give love the most they can. They might even approach this soul who was their neglected child in that former life to be born to them again as their child. And this soul out of loving readiness to help consents to be born as their child anew. And it could even be that this time it might come back as a mongoloid or handicapped child – so the parents can really prove their love for it.

   In this case the child itself often has no karma to balance, though, of course, there is also the combined case where the child has also a karmic reason to be handicapped or to possess a bodily or mental disturbance. Such a soul can also be born as a child who experiences an early death because of illness or accident. And it may not have its own karmic reasons to die early, but perhaps it is only supposed to have a certain effect on its parents, who in that way experience an act of karmic balancing or who perhaps may be pushed in this way to search for the answer to the question why "God" took away their beloved child so early.

   I have seen parents several times who were led in this

way onto the spiritual path, where they hoped to discover why this terrible event had to happen to them and why such an innocent child, who had its whole life before it, had to die so suddenly. And they found on this search for answer the way to inner spiritual truths giving them knowledge and at the same time consolation. All these events were, as we will see later, planned and arranged beforehand in the beyond in order to attain a certain learning goal.

5. **Relationship Karma** refers, as the name already implies, to relationships of all kinds: partnerships or close friendships, close acquaintanceships and family relationships – or negative relationships to employers, colleagues, employees or even other persons with whom one had no desire to associate but who crossed one's path nevertheless. Thus in every life there are confrontations with many persons with whom one has positive or negative contact and with whom one revives earlier contacts in order to carry positive or unfinished balancing programs further or even to complete them.

   We can perhaps remember the case of Mario (Case 28), who was in an earlier life the daughter of a man who sexually abused her, causing the mother to hang herself and the baby born of this incestuous relationship to be aborted. In Mario's present life this father is Mario's girlfriend, and the aborted child is their son. So Mario and his partner are involved in an intensive karmic relationship, which old karmic patterns keep popping up to disturb. But their son binds them together. The purpose of this life is for them to learn to relate to each other in genuine love, while Mario as the earlier daughter has offered himself to his partner, the earlier father, to allow him to make up for his earlier behavior. Mario himself must learn to forgive the soul of his earlier father. In this partnership, however, there are still many intertwined threads to be unraveled.

Every personal relationship is a mutual learning team. Because every incarnation is carefully planned beforehand in the beyond to attain the best "result", thus all relationships are of importance, though of varying intensity.

Because the word "karma" is primarily used in the negative sense of being met by an unpleasant event, we want here to emphasize again that karma is merely the law of cause and effect and that it also refers to positive consequences from earlier lives. But in this book, too, of course, the emphasis is necessarily on negative results, and the regression therapist is normally being consulted by clients who are suffering from negative karmic entanglements.

6. **Collective karma:** As far as I know, the first one to coin terms for social karma was Helena P. Blavatsky. After her, it was Rudolf Steiner who gave it special emphasis. Later Indian and other representatives of karmic philosophy integrated this idea into their works. Apparently, however, Buddhist thinkers had already used similar concepts in their philosophy.[54] Among

54. Zander (SW. 43) reports that in Buddhist scriptures of unknown date not only family karma but also group and national karma are mentioned.

these newly coined terms belong such concepts as "group karma", "folk karma", "race karma" and "national karma". The respective names give us a clue as to their meaning. These terms aim to point out that all sizes of groups – even up into the millions – may reincarnate together in order to make up for something that they had carried out together in a common earlier life.

To give a few examples: All the perpetrators of a planned train wreck causing the loss of many persons meet each other again "by chance" in a later life and lose their lives in another "tragic" train wreck. Or: A whole people who in an earlier life went to war with one or more other peoples, taking away all their possessions and causing the survivors to die of starvation, have to suffer together the same fate by drought or war.

I would like to take a third example from Edgar Cayce, who was responsible for an enormous improvement in the awareness of reincarnation and karma in the Western world, although his works only reached a larger public after his earthly death. The voices speaking through the mouth of this "sleeping prophet" declared that those Spaniards who participated in the slaughters during the conquest of Mexico and South America themselves had to suffer their karmic reactions by dying in the Spanish Revolution of the 1930s.[55]

There are great numbers of such karmic groups. But every member of them experiences his own personal

55. Edgar Cayce I, p. 244-252

karma. No one is forced to take part in a common group or national fate. Everyone has to have made his or her own decision to take part in such a planned action.

National karma only builds the framework for very personal karmic fates. But "interest groups" can form in the beyond in order to suffer through a common fate – for the very special reason of being able in a reincarnation to finally rid themselves of karmic burdens by together experiencing what they had done to others in an earlier incarnation (a purification process that they possibly had already been postponing for many lives -but that would be somewhat easier if experienced together).

Helena P. Blavatsky sees the karma of everyone in the context of several or even very many other persons: "Every personal misdeed of mortals is ...a double-sided sword in the hand of karma: one side for the evil-doer, the other for the family, the nation, sometimes even the race that brought him forth."[56]

7. **Karma of atonement** is very widespread and occurs in persons who have an unconscious guilt complex. This stems, unknown to them, from a life as a perpetrator in which they caused others some terrible suffering. Now they are attempting to balance this in this life by service to others. Thus physicians were perhaps military officers who sent their soldiers to the front to meet the certain death. Or they caused others to lose their lives in some other way. Those who show a so-called helper syndrome – such as many nurses,

56. Diana Dunningham Chapotin in Hanson, p. 183

social or welfare workers, even some politicians – often act for reason of a personally planned atonement program. This may appear to be almost like a straitjacket. Some do all sorts of things for others, while they neglect themselves because of their karmic program of self-punishment.

Monika (Case 16) was a Roman soldier in her life as a perpetrator, killing many persons in the cruelest manner. And she had other coarse lives as a perpetrator. In her balancing life she had to go through terrible head and back injuries, which are still felt in her present life in the form of strong head and backaches. Even before she was permanently freed from these awful disturbances by Regression Therapy she had taken up the profession of a non-medical practitioner specializing in patients with head and back injuries. She is the typical example of a person with a helper syndrome, to whom it is more important to help than to be helped by others. And as we can learn from her case and that of others, those who are subject to the helper syndrome often turn to the same area of work in which they caused so much suffering in their life as a perpetrator.

8. **Self-punishment Karma:** This is, as we have just seen, often combined with a helper syndrome of the person in question. Out of a subconscious guilt complex, he wants to be punished for misdeeds in a life as a perpetrator. For instance, if in a life as a perpetrator he was an executioner who had killed a number of people by strangulation or decapitation, he may choose in his life as a victim to have his head cut

off and at another time to be strangled to death, from which experiences constant neck pains now result. He also may not let anyone touch his neck.

But he may even want more punishment for his former misdeeds: He is perhaps miserly toward himself by not allowing himself any luxuries, by fasting, carrying out penances or taking up the life of a monk. He may not allow himself a vacation, a new suit or new car. At the same time he may have a helper syndrome, always being ready to help his neighbors. He may also seek situations where he is put in jail and can experience full punishment. Or he may lend money to others without having it returned, to which he comments, "That's my just returns!" He may possibly want to draw additional suffering upon himself by choosing a handicap unnecessary for karmic balancing reasons. And if he has bad luck, he may say, "I knew it already. That had to happen to me."

Persons who carry self-punishment karma around with them like to choose partnerships in which they have to suffer. A woman may marry for that reason a man who is an alcoholic and beats her when he is drunk. And though she knew about his bad habits before her marriage, she wanted to marry him anyway and receive the subconsciously desired punishment, which she may even provoke further by her actions.

And of course all masochists belong to the category of self-punishers. People who come in contact with them can only shake their heads in wonder at such unusual behavior. But if they were able to understand the background of such behavior – which I am making an effort to clarify here – they could offer these persons more understanding and even love, instead of stereotyping them as perverse or crazy.

9. **Rejection karma:** This and the following three kinds of karma are all connected indirectly to self-punishment karma, but each has its own distinctive program. Rejection karma has primarily to do with the life as a victim, though its roots reach back to the life as a perpetrator, too.

   A perpetrator has raped as a soldier a number of women. In his life as a victim the soul experiences now the balancing retribution - including the subconscious self-programming: "I will never again be pretty!" When this program is once engraved in the emotional body – whether after the trauma in question or only after death – then exactly this desire will take place in a following life: She is ugly, perhaps born with a crooked mouth, already unattractive as a child, got pimples at puberty etc. – so that no man proposes to her.

   A woman can for the same reason cause her own ugliness through corpulence. For this reason it is no accident that there are more fat women than men. Someone with this karma tries to keep others away, will not allow them to come close, in the subconscious intention of avoiding a repetition of that earlier experience at any price. This differs, however, from the following "self-boycotting karma".

10. **Self-boycotting karma:** One boycotts oneself to avoid the same thing happening as took place in one's previous life or lives. This type of karma can stem either from the life as a victim or directly from the life as a perpetrator. If a woman experienced in an earlier

life, after an extremely painful birth, the loss of her baby or of her own life, she may program herself with the idea: "I will never again have a baby!" And if she is reborn as a woman, she will not be able to have a child. Either she will hide herself from all men, or her body refuses to conceive or bring forth a child.

But the same thing can happen as a result of the life as a perpetrator. If a soul has smothered the child directly after birth, a similar programming can cause in the present life a "boycott of motherhood". In my book *Das große Handbuch der Reinkarnation – Heilung durch Rückführung* I report on a U.S. soldier who suddenly caught diabetes just as he was sent to the Vietnam War. So he could not be sent to the front. In fact his illness worsened to the point that he had to be discharged from the military.

In a life in about 700 A.D. he had as the leader of a mounted patrol been ordered by a sultan to completely stamp out the lives of a rebellious Christian community who refused to accept the Prophet Mohammed. Later he was plagued by his bad conscience and programmed himself with the words, "I will never again kill." This program functioned as a boycott mechanism, preventing him from being put in the position of having to kill again. I have put diabetes as well as multiple sclerosis under the heading of karmic preventive illnesses because they serve to protect their sufferers from doing something that they have decided never to do again.

But let us take a look at two more examples from the present book. The reader will surely remember Willy (Case 25), who suffered from muscular dystrophy. He was a Russian war-hero in the 16th Century, whose "hit-list" of killings was very long. His subsequent programming was: "I will never again kill." This boycott mechanism showed up in his present life as muscular dystrophy, which since his teens has kept him in a wheel chair. Now in old age he even lacks complete control over his arms. So he "does not have to kill anyone". Though in this life there was no reason for such a boycott, this program was still in effect.

The other case of self-boycott (Case 15) is one of "knife-phobia". The present Viviane was in a life as a Viking a great villain, and to make sure that this would never happen again the soul gave itself the following program: "I will never again attack anyone." In this life the manifestation of this program was chewing her nails to keep them short.

11. **False-fear karma:** Dick Sutphen[57] who was one of my teachers in Regression Therapy, coined this term for this and the next type of karma, giving the following examples: A man works day and night to insure that his family lacks nothing – he is a real workaholic! In a Regression Therapy session we find out that in an earlier life he could find no work, losing his whole family from starvation. Finally, after burying his last child with his own hands, he died himself. His program must have been: "I will never again let my family starve to death." This fear had burrowed itself deep into his subconscious, making him take on an extraordinary workload today.

57. Sutphen II, p. 41

12. **False-guilt karma:** False-guilt karma is similar to false-fear karma. Dick Sutphen relates how a man was handicapped by polio in his right leg so that he was unable to drive a car. In the Regression Therapy session he was found to have been involved in a car-accident in which a child was killed. Though he was completely innocent of wrongdoing, he took all the blame on himself. His programming: "I will never again run over a child", kept him – by means of the polio affliction in his right leg – from manipulating a gas-pedal. Such false fear or false-guilt karma can be quickly cured by taking the client to the source of his program and by dissolving it there. This can free him quickly from this complex remnant from another life.

13. **Symbolic karma:** As far as I know, Edgar Cayce first created this term. If someone was very conceited and overbearing in a previous life, he may now be hunchbacked, as a karmic reaction to help him learn humility. His present hunchback is now symbolic karma from his previous life, which he of course had chosen for himself in the beyond. Because everything that we experience in our life we have in principle already chosen voluntarily beforehand. Another example: Someone who in a previous life turned a deaf ear to the pleas of the needy and destitute may be born deaf in this life. We could also include Viviane's nail chewing (Case 15), as just described, because it is not only self-boycotting but also symbolic.

    Vera (Case 18) suffers in her present life from pains radiating from the trigeminal nerve. In an earlier life she was a very aggressive pimp, for which reason her left jaw was beaten with sticks in a life as a victim. This is the cause of her present suffering. But her Higher Self tells her that she cannot be completely healed until she overcomes her arrogance. From this viewpoint her trigeminal pains are a symbolic karma for her arrogance, which she has carried over from an earlier life.

14. **Organism karma:** This term was also coined by Edgar Cayce as an expression for the fact that bodily characteristics programmed in an earlier life may be transformed into their opposites in the present life. So someone who had programmed himself in an earlier life never to experience hunger may be fat in his present life. Often clients suffering from obesity (cf. Case 26) had starved in earlier lives and then programmed themselves never again to suffer from hunger. This transposed itself in subsequent lives into corpulence. Once the cause of this program is followed to its source, it can be cancelled and the body again gradually normalized.

15. **New Karma (Agami- or Kriyaman-Karma):** This is the name for any newly acquired karma, whether good or bad. If one desires to take good karma into his next life, he should follow the suggestions made in the chapter below: "When and how can karma come to an end?"

16. **Instant karma:** This refers to karma that I cause in this life and the reactions to which I also suffer in this life. If I steal something in this life and something is stolen from me in the same life then it could be instant

karma. Many people have experienced this often in their present lives. If one feels happy to see others involved in an accident, one can himself be involved in one in this life. The boomerang may fly back quickly!

The great Chinese master Yuen Liao Fan wrote a moral treatise in the 16th Century entitled "Four Essays On Karma", in which he shows how karma may be balanced in the same life. He even maintains that families with many children must have earned this benediction by good deeds. What appears negative in this life we have caused ourselves and can still be changed through self-knowledge. "Whoever recognizes that everyone's life is determined from inside is wise."[58] But Yuen Liao attributes balancing acts to the spirits, who can recognize precisely what one is thinking, saying and doing and can therefore bring about just karmic balancing – if possible still in this life. Therefore he warns the reader: "Do no bad deeds, for one meter above your head the divine beings are holding watch." The only way to avoid misfortune is to keep one's heart and thought pure.[59]

However, I would like to add to this the comment that instant karma can only be put into effect by higher instances if it does not conflict as a whole with the concept chosen in the beyond before the present incarnation. Usually it will not fit in, as this life is already full of other learning tasks to perform. That is one reason why ninety-five percent of the karmic reactions will be saved for the coming life or one of

58. Yuen Liao Fan: *Four Essays on Karma*, San Bruno, CA 1995, p. 22
59. Yuen Liao Fan, p. 59

the coming lives. The other reason is that the soul who has burdened itself with some karma has to first admit its mistake, and this normally only happens from the detached vantage point in the beyond. Otherwise the learning effect would perhaps be only minimal or at least not lasting enough. But the most important reason why instant karma is not usually feasible is that it is the soul itself that should decide when and where this reaction is supposed to take place. But, of course, instant karma can be put into effect if it has already been agreed upon in the beyond between the soul and the "divine beings", as Yuen Liao names them, that a balancing event is to be immediately put into effect when certain misdeeds are done.

As a whole, however, postponed karma refers mainly to major misdeeds that cannot easily be balanced or partially balanced by earthly institutions in the present life. There are even many seminars held today about the bad effect of negative thoughts, statements and deeds on our lives here and now. When we have understood this mechanism, we can greatly improve our life quality by changing our way of thinking about things, other people and ourselves.[60] Because we are the creators of our own thoughts. So we should learn to use them to form a life in which we can feel satisfied, even if there are still old karmic entanglements and patterns in effect. The law of cause and effect is also valid for small things: everything I send out comes back to me later.

60. In this connection I would like to especially recommend the books of Professor Kurt Tepperwein.

17. Stored karma (*sanchit*-karma): Everything that is inscribed in the logbook of life and that does not produce a karmic reaction in this life belongs to stored karma. Also everything that we have done up to now in this life, if it is negative, must be balanced out in one life or another. A lot of stored karma has been slumbering for many centuries without becoming active, because we have not yet included it in our presently planned itinerary for experiencing and balancing. But, as we have said, everything listed on the minus side must be balanced out sooner or later, that is, if not ... (this alternative we will save for later!).

In the meantime nice "bonus points" may also have been entered on the plus side, which of course will manifest themselves sooner or later in an earth life, too. "The abilities and insights that you attain throughout many lives are there for good. They may remain in a very hidden form. But they are biding their time, waiting for the right opportunity to be manifested in your present."[61] Dick Sutphen speaks here directly of developed ability and awareness karma.

18. Karma in the beyond: By this I mean all the accrued karma, whether good or bad, from our present life that becomes effective after death. Because that which we "sow" in a life we will "reap" already in a preliminary harvest in the beyond. As we will soon see, earthy miscreants are led after leaving this world temporarily into dark rooms or areas representing

61. Sutphen I, p. 50

symbolically their own inner life, while those who have lived a life of serving their neighbor, especially those who have finally managed to reach the end of their long path through many lives on earth, are led into the beautiful realms of the beyond. Here, too, the law of cause and effect is fully valid. Christianity and Mohammedanism have limited their concept of karma (though they do not use this term for it) to retributive justice in the beyond, where their believers are supposed to be judged according to their good or bad deeds. At least in Christianity some of the condemned are believed to have a further opportunity to balance their karma account there.

19. **Earth-bound karma:** Many souls bind themselves so much to their possessions or to things and persons that even after death they are attached to them and want to remain near them. They then do remain, in a form invisible to the physical eye, though under certain circumstances they can make themselves perceptible as "spooks" or "ghosts". Here, too, the law of free will and that of cause and effect reign. But sooner or later these earth-bound beings will also have to be led into the beyond.

These souls are sometimes able to enter into the aura or even the bodies of human beings and manipulate them or impress their own will on them. These invisible beings are not necessarily negatively poled and often wish the best for the hosts to whom they have attached themselves.

Many such "possessed" people panic and land in psychiatric clinics. But I believe that no one is haunted by accident. For, as we know, there are no accidents; here, too, law and order rule. Perhaps it is true that those haunted or possessed by one or more invisible earth-bound beings were once themselves such ghosts that now must make the same experience for karmic reasons in order to realize how much fear and suffering these beings can cause. Therefore we have to establish another category of karma, which is listed in the following: possessive karma.

20. **Possessive karma:** This was described in the previous section in connection with the earth-bound beings that haunt or possess such people for karmic reasons. Such obsessed persons may even lose control over their lives, having only little if any free will left in their thinking, speaking and acting. Sometimes persons are only temporarily or sporadically troubled by such a "companion", who however may – especially if they are under the influence of alcohol – influence them to do things that they would never think of doing in a sober condition and that may cause them considerable embarrassment or even harm. But there is sufficient secondary literature on this phenomenon.[62]

21. **Corrective karma:** This type of karmic event was already planned by the soul in the beyond and carries the following meaning: "If I still make the same mistakes from an earlier life, or other mistakes not in accordance with my plan for this life, I wish a certain thing – perhaps an accident or illness, or something like a self-boycott – to happen to me to remind me

62. See footnote 35 above, where such literature was already named.

that I have done something wrong and prevent me from taking steps in the false direction". I once had a MS-patient as a client who, as her Higher Self declared to me, had only contracted multiple sclerosis because she had again shown exactly the same arrogant behavior as in her previous life. Many of these cases of corrective karma turn up as preventive illnesses.

But a correction can also take a different form. If I am, e.g., English and have decided never to leave my homeland (except perhaps on holiday), but decide at some point to emigrate to Australia, I may be prevented forever by a sudden illness or accident from carrying out my new plan – even if I already have my ticket and a work permit in my pocket! Or a man may – after agreeing in the beyond to meet and marry a certain other soul – be fascinated by another woman and decide to marry her instead. But the second woman then may suddenly meet and fall in love with someone else. Or a soul may decide to become a nurse in its next life in order to practice humility and devotion. But, once incarnated, she may change her mind and decide to become a doctor to impress her father and gain higher prestige. But in her examinations she fails again and again despite all her effort and talents and is forced to take up the occupation she had originally planned in the beyond. The change from her original plan had to be corrected again and again, causing her tears, loss of self-confidence and depressions after every failure.

And many souls that have decided in the beyond to make their next life a spiritual one, but later become attracted to material life again, have to suffer through many aching experiences for body and soul before they enter again upon the spiritual path originally chosen but now forgotten by them. In this case we have either planned such correctional measures in detail beforehand, or requested our karma controllers to force us back on the once chosen path by all necessary means. This last type of karma is therefore not always connected with our previous life and thus it may be closer to the following "karma-free" karma.

22. **Karma-free karma:** This formulation may seem confusing, even contradictory, but actually it is quite logical. Karma-free karma stems from the fact that many things that happen in our lives are not a result of karma but still have a great influence on us. These effects are also caused, but not for karmic reasons. Like all karma, this last kind of karma is also planned in the beyond before my next incarnation. I could, perhaps, plan there for my next life – as a result of my own insight or on the suggestion of someone else – not to get a partner despite all my efforts. Because I have realized that, whether pleasant or not, I had not been able to properly appreciate my previous relationships but had taken them for granted. By experiencing the lack of a relationship, I would like to learn to value them once and for all.

    Here there is no "program" carried over from a previous life (e.g.: "I will never again have a partner."), but this decision has been made on the basis of the insight that this would be the best way to increase my ability to love. Such a life without a partner would awaken in me such longing that I would probably be more able to value one in my subsequent lives. And certainly my councilors in the beyond would praise me for having reached this decision on my own.

In this way I can fill my plan for the coming earth life with many such relevant things not chosen according to karmic considerations. So I can even choose a difficult life on earth, even e.g. blindness, because, lacking karmic grounds, I have never had the experience before. I can also decide (e.g.) to come as the mentally disturbed child of someone in order to aid him in his spiritual development – not as a sacrificial act on karmic grounds, but completely voluntarily without being predestined to do it.

Thus Jesus could also, for instance, have put together his life plan completely voluntarily, without any karmic necessity, in order to carry out a certain mission on earth. He is even, to insure its success, prepared to accept a cruel death. Or somebody plans to become a writer and decides from the beginning never to marry or have children, so that he can carry out his plan undisturbed and is not forced at any time to write whatever is presently demanded just to maintain his family. Because he would like to restrict his writing to the subjects inspired by those whom he met in the beyond and who were inspired to work together with him on a mutual literary project on earth. And he decides to enter into this project, although he knows from the beginning that it will not bring him universal approval and easy profit, but rather will entangle him in the karma-free karma processes necessary to attract public attention to his literary mission.

All this and much more belongs to karma-free karma. And some people should be tested in the alpha-state as to what in their lives stems from negative or positive karma and what stems from karma-free karma. There are still an unlimited number of things to be discovered in Regression Therapy – the treasures we have found up to now are only the beginning!

23. **Akarma:** Our list of the different types of karma would not be complete without considering also akarma (non-karma). This means that karmic misdeeds should be balanced or made up for, if possible, as soon as they have happened, so that a reaction never occurs. We can draw the following analogy: If I write a word wrong on the blackboard and immediately erase it, it is just as if I had never wrote it incorrectly. Likewise, if I commit an offense against someone in thoughts but become aware of it immediately and send him good thoughts, apologizing in my mind for my bad thoughts, then that bad thought has now been cancelled out by this good one.

    Thoughts are not nearly so strong as karmic causes as words are. If I say to someone e.g. "I could strangle you!", "I hope you have a wreck" or "I hope your wife never gives you a baby", then earnest karmic consequences could be the result. When I calm down and reflect on the consequences afterwards, I should go to the person or write him and say, "I would like to apologize for what I said then. I was so angry and got carried away. Please forgive me." Regretting one's deeds or apologizing for them can remove latent karma before it goes into effect. It is not important whether the injured person accepts the apology or not. But far stronger than the effect of thoughts or words is that of deeds. If I stick a knife out of anger into someone's arm, I will receive at some time the same or a similar karmic reaction. If I regret this act and apologize to the person or even make it up to him in some loving way, then this karmic law will no longer be valid.

But there is little use in listing here a whole catalogue of cases and the ways in which they can be neutralized. It is in the end the soul itself who decides in the beyond to what extent a karmic reaction is necessary, so that one may be kept from committing such an act again. Besides allowing us to experience the opposite situation, the law of karma serves, as we now know, to help us in our spiritual development to attain more and more love. Akarma is the canceling of a deed that otherwise would cause karma, before it can effect us in the form of a karmic reaction. The quicker one begins, the better. However, if one has committed a very bad deed though it may take a long time before one begins to regret and atone for it, one can still possibly reduce a part of its negative effects.

The deeper meaning of karma in respect to illness and suffering

Almost everyone meets with an illness or some physical disability in his or her life. When this happens we are thrown out of our life routine, forced to lie in bed or even in hospital. At this time we are dependent on the care of others – who for the reason of balancing out their own karma also need to help. Not only the ill person is involved in illness. Also the healthy person caring for him gets the opportunity not only to balance their karma but also to expand his own love, in accordance with the motto "Love your neighbor…."

In this way the ill person has a double mission: for himself and for those caring for him. This is just one example of the higher principle that everything in the world stands in a mutual interrelationship, that of course applying especially to personal relationships. For the ill person, too, there is a question of love for himself and love for others. His illness gives him, on the one hand, the chance to reflect on his own existence and on his illness. And on the other, he has an opportunity to practice patience, trust, confidence and many other virtues. He should use this opportunity to ask himself, "Why am I ill? What is actually wrong with me inside and outside?"

Because no illness just pops up by chance, there must be deeper causes over and beyond what the doctors can find. Illness is also a test. Am I angry with God, or do I recognize that I myself am the cause of this problem? Regression Therapy has proved conclusively that everyone is the source of his or her own illnesses. Everyone decides even before beginning this life what illnesses he needs for karmic reasons in order to return to himself and his love. Because in the beyond he has full awareness of what his soul needs in order to grow.

The causes for illness usually come from our own earlier lives – we cannot blame anyone else. We choose an illness in order to suffer – for fundamental and personal karmic reasons. It is thus a question of having the experience, which is at the same time connected with our inner growth.

There is also no "accidental" illness, not even a bee-sting. No one is hit "accidentally" on the head by a brick. Everything is subject to higher planning. From the cases delineated here we could clearly see that the different symptoms resulted from the different causes in lives as a victim (which again resulted from lives as a perpetrator). An illness refers us to the fact that something from an earlier life – generally at the same part of the body – needs to be investigated and cleared up. Illnesses are like fingers pointing at earlier events that are still stored in the emotional body. Of course the earlier events can also have taken place in one's present life. But my experience shows that illnesses stem in 90% of all cases from earlier lives.

And even if the cause for a grave symptom seems medically to show a clear source in the present life, this source will generally be connected to causes from earlier lives. Thus a child may catch whooping cough in kindergarten and now have a serious illness. One may then say, "What does that have to do with an earlier life? The child has obviously caught the illness from other children, just as perhaps other children in the same class have." But if the child had not had a susceptibility for such an infection there would have been none. And this susceptibility must have arisen somewhere, otherwise it would not show up. If the child for instance suffocated on smoke in an earlier life, this may have caused the susceptibility. So here, too, the law of karma is at work.

Many people see different illnesses clearly as results of genes inherited from the parents and/or grandparents, who suffered from the same problem. But if someone suffers from hemophilia and belongs to a family in which this illness has turned up repeatedly in earlier generations, this is by no means a sign that it cannot be karmic. Because if someone establishes for himself the need to have this illness in order to balance a certain karmic problem, he may choose (i.e. choose it himself or have his guides choose it for him) just such a family in which the proper genes are present.

So here too the law holds that we only take up our own inheritance, even though it superficially may seem to be otherwise. To demonstrate this we only need in a Regression Therapy session to request a hemophiliac to ask his Higher Self for an explanation why he has this illness. Immediately the karmic connections will be revealed – together with the reason why he desired to experience the illness in the given family. In the future the medical faculties at universities will have to include the subject "Karmic Etiology" (The Study of Karmic Causes) as to how and where to find the real causes. But the real point is not the discovery of karmic causes – however interesting that may be – but mainly the elimination of the symptoms or the actual healing of the illness.

And here one will often have to use Regression Therapy. Because the important thing is the uncovering of the connections leading to the symptom. The client will thus discover the cause in a life as a victim and then have to go into the life as a perpetrator. Experience will show that only then can we reach the root of the problem, leading to a high success rate and rapid healing. The patient must forgive himself in the life as a perpetrator, before forgiveness in the life as a victim can succeed. Healing means therefore: returning to the source of all causes and understanding their connections.

Healing, seen in this way, is an act of recognition and

reconciliation - centering in forgiving oneself. If we – as patients/clients – have recognized the real connections and forgiven (ourselves and others) fully, openly and without any reservations, then harmony will have been re-established and healing – as symbolic harmony formation – can take place.

Illness is an expression of karmic disharmonies that are crying for harmonization. And love is the proof-stone of harmony. Edgar Cayce described illness as an expression of sin. And sin is always an offense against love. Thus the source of all illness is callousness, i.e. loveless acts (carried out in a life as a perpetrator), whose balancing is still taking place in the present life or has already taken place in one or more lives, the symptoms in this life perhaps being only a repercussion from earlier ones.

Whatever the case may be, illnesses can be dissolved by recognition of their causality and through loving reconciliation (i.e. balancing) – if solution is already allowed. We have seen namely that the Higher Self may state that complete solution in several cases could not yet be carried out, as the karmic reactions were still necessary or other preconditions on the side of the client had to be fulfilled (cf. Case 29, where Anna still had to learn humility, und Case 18, where Vera had to rid herself of arrogance). But in any case an improvement should result already due to increased recognition and reconciliation in love.

And Tony (Case 23) recognized clearly that his psoriasis was meant to lead him to spirituality. His condition had forced him to search for the true causes and to concern himself with the topic of illness in general, leading to his giving up his original profession as a geologist and becoming a non-medical practitioner. As a result of his investigations into the original causes, he turned to spirituality, finally taking up Regression Therapy, where the actual causes for his psoriasis were revealed. Now as a regression therapist he is helping others to discover the causes of their illnesses, in order to heal themselves by recognition and reconciliation.

Illness serves the expansion of love and awareness, with its final aim being spiritual salvation. Because he who heals himself within also contributes to saving our world. In the alpha-state Liane (Case 12) transmitted deep truths on the subject "suffering", which she received from an old wise man in the beyond. Suffering belongs, as he said, to the universe. All beings, whether they are humans, animals etc., want to suffer, for this belongs to their independence. These statements will arouse protest in almost every intelligent person. But if we consider what we have already heard in this book about original karma – i.e. our decision from the standpoint of higher intelligence before entering the material plane to experience the opposite of divine harmony in the form of a stone, plant, animal and/or human – then we may be able to understand what the wise-man was trying to tell Liane. And it will also make his next statement understandable, namely that karma is the result of our wish to suffer, our particular karma even being personally chosen by us.

It was thus our own higher decision to accept karma, together with the suffering that comes along with it. We have to get used to seeing things from a higher perspective, if we are to see the central aspects of life in their true light. We have to get to the bottom of earthly life, seeing it in its relativity – something only possible if we are used to perceiving it also from the perspective of other, higher realities. Only then can we see the law of karma in its actual perfection. And the old man also said that suffering is the pre-condition for all development – that it was through suffering that we reached love.

These statements could perhaps inspire the modern reader to meditate about them by closing his eyes and reflecting on these points in connection with similar statements that I have often hinted at here. And if one also goes deep within, asking in meditation for further explanations on this theme, it is possible that one may receive telepathic answers from "above" – something that happened e.g. to the author Neale Donald Walsch, leading him to write a series of best-sellers under the title "Conversations with God".

Fate and destiny as karma

Out of respect for the great philosopher Plotinus – to whom I have also devoted a proper place in my Caesarian drama *Valerian* – I would like to give the reader in the following a sampling of his thought. Upon reading his works, I was astounded to discover that most of the secrets that we have uncovered in the course of Regression Therapy were already mentioned in his works (as compiled by his disciple Porphyrios in the *Enneads)*:

"Furthermore, that which we have called here 'unjust' is not an evil for the one who must suffer it, because it perhaps contributes to the totality of his plan. Or it is not at all unjust, being justified by earlier lives offenses. One should not believe that only a part of the events are predestined and the other part left to free choice. Because if everything is supposed to work according to the causes and effects of a unified plan and a unified order, then the more insignificant events must also be included and integrated in this plan.

"Therefore also the mentioned 'unjust' acts done by one person to another are certainly injustices for the doer himself – who thus is not relieved of guilt. They are however an integral part of the whole chain of events, and therefore in this total framework they are no injustice. Also they are no injustice to him who suffers them, but were determined to be carried out against him, and if the sufferer is good in his thoughts then the bad things done to him amount to something good in the end account.

"Because one must not call this law (karmic law) ungodly and unjust, but only extremely exact in the distribution of its appropriate application. Its ways remain also hidden, so that for us who do not understand them it seems to offer cause for complaint."[63]

The fate of a human is subject to a total plan constructed in the *Nous* (which should be imagined as a spiritual station for projecting new worlds and souls to populate them) and is as an integral part of this plan also important for the whole. Within this plan the free will of the individual has its radius of movement, and everything suffered on earth also is part of this plan. Everything is so ordered that even apparent trivialities are significant.

From the viewpoint of the total plan a perpetrator does no evil deeds – but from an earthly standpoint this is different. And we may remember what was said about the experience of the opposite of the divine all-harmony and all-love. Because Plotinus touches directly on this point. On the earthly level also the sufferer experiences no

63. Plotinus, Enneads, *Problems of the Soul, I*, §§ 86 ff. (in Harder, p. 205f.)

injustice, it being already pre-determined for him on karmic grounds. And that which he suffers is even good, as it frees him of a karmic burden – if he now remains virtuous and avoids burdening himself with further karma.

Now the great words full of philosophical depth: "...one must not call this law ungodly...". Because everything is measured exactly, even though its justification is not apparent to us and we are not able to understand its higher meaning.

At another place Plotinus, who does not use the word *karma*, says, "The fate of the individual is inseparable from his past and his future. Everyone has created the cause in an earlier life of his present fate and is now preparing his future fate."[64] No one can escape, he goes on to say, "what he is accorded to suffer because of his improper deeds", for "the divine law is inescapable".[65]

A human being is subject to the inevitable law of karma for which he himself is responsible. Whoever is met by illness, poverty, oppression or any other such fate has assigned this fate to himself. Not God but the individual person himself is responsible. Each fate is exactly allotted; nothing is unjustified. Thus our fate mirrors our deeds.

From one's fate it is often possible to deduct one's former deeds, something a regression therapist should be able to do well, since he has already had a lot of experience in this area. Fate is also the teacher making us aware of the mistakes that we have made in the past. Because everything that separates us from God or unity is negative and requires karmic balancing in order to re-establish harmony. And everything that brings us closer to

64. Quoted in Kafka, p. 247
65. Harder, p. 223

God, the all-harmony and all-love is positive.

We are the creators, the bearers and also the conquerors of our fate.[66] "It is not fate that makes our lives difficult but the decisions that we have made and whose consequences we are now experiencing as karma. In order to overcome karma we have to return to the decisions we have made and erase these consciously."[67] This is a process that can best be carried out through Regression Therapy.

Since everyone experiences his own individual pre-established fate, no one dies a death that is not pre-determined. And, as experience has shown, a bullet hits the person whose karma it is to receive it often exactly at the place where he killed someone else in an earlier life. The reader can probably remember Uwe, the doctor with the heart condition (Case 21). He had as a French officer jabbed his rapier into the heart of his already helpless dueling-opponent. In his life as a victim as a French soldier in 1914, he was hit directly in the heart by a bullet while on the front, of which the heart cramps in his present life are a repercussion.

And this brings up the question as to what invisible powers intervene to guide one bullet among thousands so that it hits no one else but the person for which it is meant – and in fact exactly at the pre-established place. So we must be accompanied by invisible beings guiding the events

---

66. This sentence has been taken from the notes for Professor Kurt Tepperwein's training seminars *Ausbildung zum Lebensberater* (Training of Life counselors) which he gives every year in Switzerland. His knowledge on the topics reincarnation and karma is documented in his book *Schicksal und Bestimmung*, which is one of the most important books for expansion of spiritual consciousness.

67. Vallières, p. 114

according to our very special karma. Nothing happens by chance; everything is planned. Such invisible helpers belong to a specially trained group of persons in the beyond guiding our fate according to the pre-established plan. They act exactly in accordance with the law of karma.

They are incorruptible, arranging everything necessary to fulfill the karma that we have set by our deeds, bad and good. These "karma-managers" or "karma-arrangers", as one could call them, make sure that a bullet does not hit someone by accident for whom it is not intended. It is certainly a great art – especially in a hail of bullets – to arrange the events so that they only hit those who are preordained to receive them. They also see to it that in a train wreck only those so predestined are killed or injured there. And if only one person is predetermined to survive in a plane crash, they will make all arrangements to ensure that he or she somehow gets through.

There is a so-called "law of karmic resonance" according to which only those persons are subject to a certain fate who carry the specific resonance in them. And this resonance is based on their karmic disposition. So, for instance, in a deadly explosion those persons survive or remain unhurt who had no resonance for death or injury, while all those who possessed the proper resonance for death had to die. Or another example: A woman for whom no rape experience was planned could go into the forest and see men for whom this might be a "good opportunity" and still remain unmolested. A different woman, for whom such a rape as a karmic reaction was to be expected, could quite well be raped if she went alone into the forest. In the same way air-travelers may be kept for inexplicable reasons from taking a certain flight because they are not fated to die in the impending plane-crash. Some may say "pure accident" – but this doesn't exist. Religious people speak in such cases of divine intervention or of their guardian angel.[68]

In the longest novel of German literature ever written, I have related the fate of the German people in the years 1933-1949, describing their karmic connections. Because I applied the law of karma to all the persons involved I was even taken to court, resulting in the third (of four) volumes – entitled *Jedem das Seine* ("To Each His Own") – at present still being forbidden for sale in Germany.[69] In the fourth part, *Maria*, the time of the two World Wars was described as the greatest period of karmic balancing in history. During the period of the Second World War alone, approximately a hundred million persons lost their lives – many in the most brutal way. In all, about one billion persons were directly or indirectly affected, and millions of them suffered from hunger, destitution, exile, loss of relatives, injury, loss of limbs, loss of possessions, etc.

Millions of souls wanted their debits finally erased from their account before the beginning of a new millennium. Because they wanted to incarnate and pursue their spiritual development in this new age with as little "karmic baggage" as possible. This was preceded in the beyond by a gigantic collective campaign to finally clear up all those debits through this experience of karmic balancing. The people of

68. Edgar Cayce allows however that in creation itself accidents and chance occurrences are quite possible. Cerminara, p. 248
69. The four volumes appearing separately were *Molar* (this volume can be read in Internet in a full seven-color version uncondensed under *www.trutzhardo.com*), *Lilia, Jedem das Seine* and *Maria.* Three of these volumes are available in Silberschnur Verlag (*www.silberschnur.de*). My court case on karma can be reviewed in Internet, *www.bhakti-yoga.ch/hardo.*

today do not have enough distance to these events yet to realize what gigantic karmic proportions they reached.

But where is there free will? To clarify that I will use an analogy I would like to call the "train of fate": At my birth a long railway-train stops in front of me. I get in. I have a reserved seat determining whether I have a pleasant window-seat, a seat near the door (where the cold wind attacks me) or even have to sit pressed in the middle between two heavy neighbors. All these things are pre-established, but also who will be riding with me in the compartment and for how long.

But I myself still do have the free will to decide how I will behave in this compartment, whether I – while sitting in a non-smoking compartment – without asking anyone's permission thoughtlessly light up my cigar, or whether I pull out my sweets and enjoy eating them all by myself before the eyes of wide-eyed children, or if I observe an old lady as she pulls a heavy suitcase from the luggage rack, hoping secretly that it will offer me some private amusement by falling on her head. These things happen out of my own free will, bringing about future karmic reactions for me.

The coordinates for the life in my "train of fate" are already set. I have no freedom of decision now concerning the already pre-established train and seat numbers, fellow-passengers and the time of entering and leaving the train, as they happen according to my own higher insight and in alignment with my own free will and earlier choice in the beyond.

In my voluntary "new" actions within the framework of my present life, however, I still have complete freedom – although these actions are of course partly conditioned by habits and predispositions carried over from earlier lives.

Within these limits I have absolute freedom in what I think, say and do, as the results of my free decisions will only be presented to me later. But my behavior within these coordinates is already preparing the set-up for my next life.

The meaning of karmic relationships and partnerships

As we have seen in respect to the cases described here, the souls with whom we are brought together are often those we already know from earlier lives. Usually they will be previous or present family members reappearing again and again in quite different constellations. As we will see later, they generally all belong to the same internal group in the beyond, whose members have agreed beforehand to take over specific roles while helping each other in mastering certain tasks in the "school of life". Our experience in Regression Therapy has shown that some clients have had several or even many lives with their present partner or with other close relatives etc. It seems to be a "rule" that we have to come together with certain others until all our "differences" have been resolved.

If a man of 1900 had on the average only one wife – and one job and home – in his life, we can say that this number has certainly tripled in the meantime, so that today an average man has three different jobs, three homes at different times and three long, intensive partnerships (or marriages). We can learn faster today, i.e. we are on the average confronted in all with three partners and – a partnership being also always a partnership for learning – thus have three partnership learning programs to absolve in one lifetime. As soon as we are finished our "study course" in the first partnership, we are freed for the next partnership.

That doesn't mean that we are completely finished with the first course. Usually we have made some progress already and will meet with our first partner again in our next life to continue work on our disharmony problems – until we can relate completely to each other in love. Very often the first partnership ends in a fiasco. Also the second partnership leaves a lot of room for improvement. In the third partnership often something like harmony is reached.

But sometimes a person marries repeatedly other persons with the same problem constellation. This is a sure sign that the person had decided definitely to clear up just this problem in this life, while the different partners have probably offered to be of assistance in this effort. Women often also marry someone who is a carbon copy of their father, especially in his bad sides. This too is a sign that one has in particular to work on these problems.

But divorce doesn't ever mean "forever". On the contrary, divorce is always a guarantee that they will meet in the beyond again to arrange another attempt to work out their relationship in another life time, solve their problems and attain harmony once and for all.

Every close relationship is a karmic relationship in its positive as well as its negative aspects. The learning goal is obligatory: learn to love your partner like yourself. Often such karmic relationships have begun in a terrible way, i.e. by one of the partners having killed the other in an earlier life. This was demonstrated in Case 28, in which still today – after ten further lives together – there are still areas of conflict, though they are coming closer by developing more and more love for each other, life after life.

Let us clarify this process of a "karmic relationship" with an example as follows:

Let's say the soul "X" was married to the soul "Y" around 1000 A.D. X then kills his wife Y in jealousy after discovering that Y had entered into a secret relationship with someone else. The soul Y then stored X in its emotional body as "100% negative".

Around 1200, after spending the following life with other partners, they again meet. X is now the father and Y the daughter. They will recognize each other subconsciously by the specific vibrations that remain unchanged throughout different incarnations. X will have realized the mistake he made – in the beyond, at latest – and will try subconsciously to make up for it in this life by being a good father. But again and again he is plagued by sudden attacks of anger over his wife's deception of him in their earlier life.

Y on the other hand is very much afraid of her father and will not be able to trust him, as she subconsciously remembers being killed by him in that earlier life. But she also has a bad conscience because she deceived him in their earlier life together. She wants at all costs to make up for her earlier act. She accepts therefore all of his demands, if only to avoid a similar fate in this life. There are many periods of tension between them, but sometimes there are also loving moments, and after this life Y has retained only seventy percent of her negative attitude toward X.

Two hundred years later (c. 1400) they again come together again on earth. This time Y is the father and X is his son. Y's mistrust of X is still there, causing him to dislike his son. The son tries however to please his father and is even able to save him from a burning house. Therefore Y is now indebted to X, reducing his rejection to forty percent.

About three hundred years later they again meet. This

time the soul Y is the wife of X, who still mistrusts her subconsciously. Y is faced with the same temptation as in her life in 1000 A.D., but decides to remain faithful to her husband for some subconscious reason. X gains then more and more confidence in his wife. Although there are conflicts once in a while, they also often hug each other affectionately. Soul Y feels now soul X's affection for her and can almost completely trust him. There are only minimal reservations of about five percent left.

Three hundred years later, after having in the meantime lived as two brothers and as a brother and sister, they come together again as husband and wife. Now they perhaps are able to experience for the first time living together as a pair in a harmonious relationship, which gradually becomes a deep love for each other.

When two souls have finally learned everything they can from each other, there is no conclusive reason for them to waste their precious time further with each other. Because there are certainly other souls with whom they have many things still to clear up. And because each life is precious, there is all the more reason to use them to the best possible advantage. Thus such partners need no longer to come together in close contact but may only occasionally and briefly see each other in passing. They will recognize each other immediately as souls and feel their love for one another, but respect the fact that they each have other relationships to carry out now. But in the beyond, those who have developed a close band of love will meet each other again and again, enjoying to the full their mutual inner attraction and love from soul to soul.[70]

70. Such a case of mutual loving enjoyment by two lovers in the beyond is described in my novel *Der Blinde Dichter (The blind Poet)*.

Each is the mirror of the other. Each can recognize the advantages and disadvantages in the other, supporting or restricting his further development. We will only progress on our own path if we recognize more and more our own self in our partner. Everything that I do to another I have really done to myself, for I am my other – my "alter ego". We are all one. A partnership then becomes a learning step experienced on the way to this revelation.

Karmic partnership, as well as any other interpersonal relationship, is the best "sandpaper" – used to rub each other as long as it takes to smooth off all unevenness and produce out of us perfect, shining souls. Partners are also the best mirrors to show us our own faults. The final aim is for our individual egos to find the way to "us". This is the aim of every karmic partnership, no matter how long – whether a hundred or a thousand years – it takes to discover the "we" in "I + I" as the preliminary step to final reunion with the all-love. Usually the female partner is the soul leading the male more and more toward love. Because expansion of love is her main spiritual task in respect to her partner. Therefore it is often so that during the preparations in the beyond for a new earthly life the soul that is to incarnate as a man will search for a female partner who is ahead of him in respect to love. The male principle is "educated" so to speak "in love" by the female principle. This is about what Goethe meant to say by ending his "Faust" with the words, "The eternal female principle leads us on."

Dying and death as a karmic event

When a person senses that death is nearing, he may meet this fate in various different ways. Some people are afraid of this great unknown factor that they have tried to avoid thinking of so long. Many people only occupy themselves with this subject when they are forced to, e.g. when they are extremely ill and have to take into consideration the possibility of dying. Then many suddenly have a bad conscience, for they think perhaps of all the things they have done wrong in their lives or all the people they still have "unfinished business" with. That great expert on death Elisabeth Kübler-Ross refers us to the fact that it is never too late – whether as a dying person or as the relative of one – to take care of mutually unfinished business before death, even if one only says, "Please forgive what I have done to you."

Believers in the church are afraid of a final judgment that may condemn them for their sins to eternal tortures in "Hell" – which latter, let us state that here, doesn't exist, unless one makes one's own hell. "Hell" was a great gift to the clergy, who used this idea to frighten and subject people, though it was often also a useful whip to frighten people from carrying out evil deeds.

On the whole one could say that those who are afraid of death and therefore do not want to "let go" are those who feel subconsciously that they have not completed the tasks they have set out to do. And those who are able to die in peace are the ones who are generally satisfied with themselves and their lives, for they know subconsciously that they have completed, if not all, then at least most of their plan.

Before their life on earth they had already planned themselves what they wanted to do. And it is at least better to stand up before others as someone who had again accomplished only little or nothing of his plan than to have to shamefully admit to himself and his Higher Self, "I have again failed miserably and have even committed great offenses against love." Teachers, judges, masters in the beyond are very understanding toward the returning souls despite the numerous mistakes that they have possibly made on earth. But we are generally not so tolerant toward ourselves. This fear of self-denigration is perhaps present as a subconscious undertone during the five potential phases of death.

Death is only a pause in the long life of the human soul, beginning with one's first birth as a human and ending with one's last earthly life. Every life is, as we have already mentioned, only a school day in the school of life on earth, where one is constantly confronted with the law of karma and is presented again and again love as one's main subject of study. And like the poet Novalis we could reverse the usual way of looking at things by saying, "When we are born, we die, and when we die, we are born." If we see life after death as the truer and more wonderful life – whereas life on earth is, like a school day, just difficult and strenuous period – then we surely can agree with his statement. It all depends on the perspective from which one sees things. And the higher the position is from which we gain our perspective, the more we will be able to view them in their true form.

We are talking here about the expansion of our consciousness, something that I also, for example, as an author of belletristic and non-fictional literature as well as a regression therapist and seminar-teacher wrote in my life plan – of course already before entering my present life. But proper expansion of consciousness can only be paired with expansion of love, otherwise one will be caught in false perspectives – however elevated their aim may be.

As was demonstrated in most of the cases described here, I always ask my clients in a session before or after they experience a former death how they would end the sentence "I will never again...." They may answer then, for instance, "I will never again be so callous" (Case 13), "I will never again cheat others" (Case 17), "I will never again send so many people to their deaths" (Case 9), "I will never again hurt my wife" (Case 7) or "I will never again give false witness" (Case 8).

These "never again" sentences are the statements of perpetrators at the end of or after their lives. At this time one programs him/herself – usually accompanied by remorse or repentance for one's deeds – for what one wants at all costs to avoid doing wrong again. The cause was the deed itself. The first consequence was repentance together with a "never-again" programming. The second consequence takes place in the beyond with still deeper remorse combined with the desire to make up for one's deed. The third consequence arises during planning of one's next life or lives, whereas the fourth consequence takes place in the next lives in the form of balancing the deed as a victim.

If the original programming was e.g. "I will never again kill", this can also have an effect even into the tenth consecutive life, making the client refuse military service etc. Such "never again" statements from lives as a perpetrator already point to behavior in subsequent lives. But, due to the terrible suffering experienced there, such statements turn up more commonly in, or especially after, lives as a victim.

One of these, for instance, was, "I will never again speak in public" (Case 10), after the client as a Greek orator was thrown off the cliffs for speaking too openly. In this case the details of his death were also imprinted on his emotional body, making him afraid of heights. Death is thus the most important collection-point for subsequent karmic behavior patterns.

Or we can remember the case of Rudi (Case 14), whose obsession with cleanliness stemmed from his life as a cardinal with a sexually transmitted disease, resulting in the program, "I will never again have sexual contact." And this program still had the effect in his present life of preventing all sexual relationships. Because while planning his present life it did not occur to him to change or eliminate this program, something he can now do through Regression Therapy.

As our third example we can refer to the boy who was trampled to death by cows (Case 16), resulting in the program, "I will never again act independently. I will never again overstep my boundaries." And as a result Monika still has headaches today, together with an inferiority complex.

Death as our collection-point for karmic behavior patterns registers everything connected with death or dying in our emotional body, which then becomes the carrier for all those apparently insignificant patterns as troublesome accompaniments in our daily life – if they have not already been carefully eliminated in the beyond. If one experiences death with a clear consciousness and, if possible, without pain, then one should consider what should consciously be programmed, because the next life often begins with exactly the same programs that we set up in the moment of death.

But death and dying are already karmic processes. Because everyone dies at the time pre-established by or for him in the beyond. And the process of dying together with the amount of suffering is also pre-established. As we have already variously emphasized, nothing is based on chance. There is no place in this wonderfully constructed creation for chance. Many cases of e.g. sudden death have occurred for karmic reasons, something vividly demonstrated by most of the victims' deaths described in the present book. The kind of such a victim's death or the process of his dying experienced is approximately the same as the death he/she had brought about for someone else in an earlier life.

But a long illness could also be prescribed for oneself, e.g. in order to learn humility or patience. Everything has a meaning, and uncovering the true deeper significance of karmic events is an interesting task. It is a gigantic puzzle, and I hope I have been able to connect some of the pieces. But there is still an infinite amount to do in order to view the puzzle as a whole.

Death takes place at the pre-established hour and not a second earlier. Every moment of death is exactly pre-calculated, just as the moment of birth – aside from very seldom cases of (intentional) last minute changes. In general our time runs out when our previously planned program is completed. That can be at the age of one, of ten or of a hundred. Whenever death comes, it is the right moment. Possibly the soul said to itself in the beyond before entering a life, "I will only stay twenty-five years on earth, so I can get back as soon as possible to my friends and learn some more here of what I enjoy the most." Death is only the end of the school day, returning home, relaxation and rest, reunion with relatives and friends, time for homework and preparation for the next school day.

There is an infinite amount we could say about all these things, but unfortunately this book has a set size-limit. So I must apologize to the reader who is curious to know more. But now let us take a brief look at what happens in the beyond – from the karmic side.

Temporary balancing of karma in the beyond

Shortly before our last breath we gradually begin to leave our earthly body together with our astral body, and suddenly we can see with our the eyes of our astral body. And what we see generally fills us with great pleasure. This pleasure can often be seen on the lips and in the face of the earthly body we leave behind to our folks left behind. Because we will usually be met by the loved ones preceding us into the beyond or perhaps by our female or male spirit guide who led us invisibly during our life on earth.

At this point what I have called "karma in the beyond" takes hold. For, if I have managed to demonstrate on earth a halfway positive and loving behavior, my reception in the beyond will also be very loving. Many other souls will joyfully come to greet me and congratulate me for my successful life. And if someone was able to carry out their life with bravura, spreading love everywhere, as e.g. Albert Schweitzer was able to do, then a great festival will be his reception, in which dozens, hundreds or even thousands of souls will take part.

But someone who has lived a life empty of love, perhaps having been cruel to humans or animals, can expect no reception. Possibly only his spirit guide will meet him, without any joyful hugs or heartfelt welcome, leading him then into spheres just as loveless outside as this newcomer is inside. He will be brought together in dark surroundings with others of his kind, so that they can serve each other as mirrors, thus helping each other to recognize the reasons for their callousness and cruelty.

But with the passage of time (which only exists there subjectively, not objectively) they experience a gradual brightening of their surroundings paralleling the gradual increase in their repentance and remorse.[71] Finally they reach, as Michael Newton puts it,[72] an "intensive care unit", where they are confronted with their actions in their previous life on earth. Once there, they will normally recognize and accept the law of karma and gladly be ready to balance their misdeeds by experiencing themselves exactly what they have done to others out of callousness. They then very readily accept the possibility of entering a new incarnation and leave it up to the "karma-experts" to work out a fate for them to experience in their next life something similar of what they have done unto others – to which they also easily agree.

In Case 21 the murderer is met in the beyond by the murdered rival, who greets him and readily forgives him. After a short orientation period there is no vengeance there. Because there love is practiced in perfection, and forgiveness is the trademark of love. (We enter earthly life so we can practice active love under the especially unfavorable conditions there.)

The law of karma offers the repentant the chance to correct their misdeeds. Christianity sees as its main

---

71. Allan Kardec says "that there are no sins which cannot be atoned for somewhere". For "man can find the way to atonement in different existences, paving the way for him to perfection according to his own wishes and efforts", until he has reached his final goal (Hummel, p. 80). It is astounding how Kardec already had received in the 19th century from spirits via mediums many of the basic truths later discovered by reincarnation therapy.

72. Newton, I . p. 49 und II, p. 3

formula: "God's mercy and Jesus' blood save us from our sins". But in Regression Therapy I see clearly that I myself have to make up for the damage I have done. I myself carry the responsibility for my acts. I should not depend on God's and Jesus' already having forgiven me, so that "I don't have to worry anymore about the salvation of my soul." The law of karma is God's act of mercy, leaving me the free decision to take care of my salvation myself.

"There above," says the apparently omniscient Plotinus correctly[73], "the soul finds itself in the company of those who are similar." And it is really that way. On earth we have to live in a melting pot of all different soul-vibrations, but there in the beyond we are sent to levels in accordance with our individual vibrations. Those who have lived a relatively good or even loving life are met by those of their own kind and led to the areas reserved for them. In Case 6 a young man who had a speech defect on earth and was picked on and finally beaten to death because of it was met in the beyond by his mother, who was carrying a bouquet for him. He was then led by her to his group. The daughter (Case 28) who aborted her child was met joyfully in the beyond by the child and her parents. And die raped Polish girl, Marianca (Case 2), discovered that in the beyond she was met everywhere with happy smiles – she even found laughing seemingly to be the main activity of the inhabitants there.

If someone has just experienced a terrible or difficult death, he is allowed first of all to convalesce in a sanatorium or at an especially beautiful and peaceful spot. Everything there is about ten times more beautiful than on earth.

73. Harder, p. 199

We experience the beyond every time as if it were the first time, for at this renewed entering we still have no memory of earlier lives. Our first task will be to reconsider the life just finished. But there is a more fundamental reason for our "forgetfulness". If we returned to the beyond as to something well known, our astonishment about the wonders of "heaven" would not have the same effect.

If we contact those in the beyond in séances, we may find that some of them even deny that there is reincarnation. Because souls recently arrived there who were strict followers of some religious dogmas on earth are allowed to retain their beliefs – no one is forced to accept any way of thinking, as experience will lead even these souls sooner or later to the basic truths.[74]

---

74. A part of our soul, as Plotinus also knows (Harder, p. 145), remains in the beyond. This statement is also confirmed by the researcher of the beyond Michael Newton, „Part of our light-energy always remains in the beyond" (Newton II, p. 2) . And we remember that Buddha denied the existence of a soul and therefore also reincarnation as such. He believed, as Osho interprets him (p. 145), that the thoughts of a person at death are transferred to a new child in the womb of a pregnant woman, i.e that there is no rebirth of the person himself to whom the thoughts originally belonged. And Osho – after giving many opposing views - agrees with this statement, saying that also the person remembering earlier lives are simply carrying the thoughts of other, no longer existent souls, which they interpret as thoughts of their own from earlier lives. These thoughts remind us naturally of those of C.G. Jung, who attributes such memories of earlier lives to a collective subconscious of all the thoughts ever conceived in the world.

A completely new variation of reincarnation is given by Pierre de Forêt in his extremely interesting book *Die Geburt der Seele (The birth of a soul)*. Here he expresses the idea – given to him by his spirit guide – that a soul cannot incarnate and thus no reincarnation is

Recommendable books on the beyond are those of Anthony Borgia and Michael Newton. We may remember the descriptions of Rose (Case 20) of her experiences in the beyond after she had, as a desperate priest, jumped from a church tower. The priest found himself first in a room with a dome where a waterfall was splashing into a pool. He was allowed to sit and convalesce for a while, until suddenly a light-beam from above entered his body, filling him with blissful higher knowledge.

Some newcomers are led first before judges in colored or white robes. In Case 29 they tell the murderer standing before them that he will have to be murdered himself once for each of his many victims. And the man who killed his daughter and then hanged himself is informed by the judges about his mistaken actions. Asked by his soul-guide if he is willing to clear his mistake by allowing a similar balancing reaction against himself, he agrees immediately.

---

possible. Instead, according to him, one can experience aspects of oneself in bodies now living on earth. But at death the body decomposes, and the soul can decide to have another body manifest some of one's aspects (de Forêt, p. 70f.). As interesting as all these ideas may be – and new ideas always aid the growth of knowledge – they seem to me to be illogical or too simplistic, since, as Stevenson has proved, children who remember earlier lives sometimes have birthmarks clearly reminiscent of the cause of death - which they also remember. And all of our experiences with reincarnation therapy show that the many symptoms of the clients regularly point to specific earlier lives as a victim. And all the resulting connections form a logically consistent whole. Furthermore – and this is the most convincing argument for me – their symptoms usually disappear almost immediately as soon as their earlier lives are „cleared", i.e. the causes are recognized, the law of karma is accepted as being just and reconciliation and resolution are effected.

As Michael Newton – the most extensive researcher of the beyond through Regression – describes in his extremely valuable books, many of these souls don't learn about the law of karma until these judges inform them. When Karla (Case 26) entered into the beyond after being burned as a witch, she saw, instead of a judge, a shining throne before her, where she was told that she had had to suffer this fate because of her previous life as a torturer who threw people into the flames. The scenery in the beyond accommodates itself to the way of thinking of the newcomers.

In the beyond a soul experiences first a reaction to its earthly way of thinking, speaking and acting: it is met in the way it would expect according to its earthly behavior and is led into spheres resonating in accordance with its own inner life on earth. As the procedures are chosen to fit the bad or good behavior of their earthly faring, a typical karmic pattern of cause and effect is also evident there. But everyone eventually returns to his own individual group, the one he was already in before his incarnation.

The revision of our actions on earth and karmic preparation for our next reincarnation

Michael Newton discovered that such a group usually consists of three to twenty-five members, and this agrees also with my experience. So we can speak of an average size of fifteen members.[75] These groups are composed of souls that we have already known for a long time, and we have met each other often within these groups either in the beyond or in different incarnations on earth. Some of them are very close to us, having possibly already been lovers or

75. Newton II, p. 4

close family members. We often offer our assistance to others when they want to learn different lessons in the earthly school – all of which, in the last analysis, have to do with the main subject "Love" and one or a few of its subcategories.

Every group is equipped with at least one teacher, generally masculine, who discusses very extensively the past life of every member in front of the group. All of the situations on earth in which we have brought love into play or demonstrated lack of love are projected on a kind of screen, so that all present can learn from the events exhibited. Nothing is covered up. And we ourselves become our most brutal critics.

I would like to demonstrate on a minor example how such a group carries out its work: One member of the group, whose previous life is now being discussed before the group by means of thought projections onto the "screen", discovers himself in a supermarket where he is just getting his change given back by the cashier. Outside he counts it and finds that he has received one biger bill too many with the change. And now he has a double consciousness: he remembers exactly what he was thinking at that moment and at the same time and he is momentarily ashamed of how he reacted – instead of giving it back, he kept it. Here he got a "negative load" of karma and will likewise have to make up for this mistake by being a victim of theft.

But the film continues: On the same evening the cashier has to present the final balance with the proceeds for the day to her boss. Asked about the missing sum, the cashier turns red in embarrassment, which is interpreted by the boss as a sign that she has stolen the money. He fires her in anger. The next picture: The young woman is at home, where one of her four children has contracted polio and the father is out of work and has turned to drink. Now that she, the only bread-winner in the family, has also lost her job, she sees no way to feed the family, takes in her desperation an overdose of sleeping tablets and dies.

Now his shame is all the greater when he sees all the problems he has caused. He may cry uncontrollably and regret his stupidity a thousand times. Others in the group may also think of similar cases on earth where they misused the situation to the disadvantage of others. And after the connections have been discussed, the same situation will be acted out in role-play, this time demonstrating the proper behavior.

These groups serve then to educate the souls as to the wrong actions by which they have burdened themselves with karma. And they serve to clarify proper behavior and practice. Certainly the "candidate" will meet the same situation in his next life, too. And if he puts the money in his own pocket once more, he again will be confronted in the beyond and in his group with his behavior, until he has passed all tests on earth clearly and without faltering. As mentioned above, our accompanying leaders and teachers have unbelievable patience with us. There are always slow and fast learners. That is true everywhere.

And many souls, whose words and deeds are shown to them again, are ashamed of their egoistic and loveless behavior (as in Case 2) or are happy when they have acted according to the guidelines of love. Not only are the mistakes thoroughly discussed, but also the question of how the "candidate" could have acted properly is extensively delved into. Proper behavior is then acted out in role-plays in which all the members of the group take part enthusiastically.[76] And everyone there is confronted with the law of karma, knows what he has done wrong and is prepared to enter a new incarnation in the "school of suffering and purification"[77] in order to experience the same thing that he has caused others to live through (cf. Case 2).

But this life in the beyond should not be understood as consisting only of constant group training. Besides this, there are many other very pleasant activities to occupy one's time: spending time in libraries, taking part in certain festivities, occupying oneself with long neglected hobbies, learning to play a musical instrument or taking part in research projects. And one can also invisibly return to earth, perhaps even accompanied by one's teacher while he points out on certain people's behavior. This may be useful either as a learning preparation for one's next reincarnation or for gaining an impression of how and when events planned for this reincarnation will be initiated "from above". But in this case – as an invisible being - one is not allowed to interfere in the thoughts and life of human beings unless there is good reason to do so and it is therefore authorized by higher beings.

It is easy to keep occupied in the beyond because everything is very pleasurable and interesting. Actually we humans on earth should envy our recently deceased relatives for now having ended their work on earth and being allowed to enjoy the pleasures of the beyond again! But this beyond is not only there to allow for relaxation or

---

76. Newton II, p. 193f
77. This is what Allan Kardec names the earth. (quoted in Hummel, p. 80)

for investigation of one's previous life. It is also meant as a period of preparation for the coming incarnation, which we will gladly enter as soon as we understand its purpose and its necessity. At a certain point we will see that it is necessary as a testing ground to see if we can also put that what we have learned in the beyond into practice under the much harder conditions of earthly life.

But the most important phase for the arrangement of all events on earth comes just before one's new incarnation. The soul has freedom of choice and is allowed sufficient use of it before entering upon a new life on earth. "Karma itself does not write the manuscript for the next lesson. It only lays down the framework that must be abided by. We write the curriculum ourselves together with our teachers. But the final responsibility lies always with us, as we have the right to reject any suggestion."[78] Symbolically speaking, we glance in our karmic bank account book and can see there exactly what negative karma we have to balance out for learning reasons and also what lesson we can add on as an "option" in our earthly "schoolroom".

If we are very ambitious and want to balance a lot of the karma from earlier lives, then we will choose a hard life, possibly with many misfortunes and situations where we experience just the treatment ourselves that we have hard-heartedly dealt out to others before. Even the ex-murderer is ready, after his period of repentance and his experience in his soul-group, to recognize the law of karma and accept his karmic lot in a new life. Yes, he will even be happy to grasp the opportunity to erase the earlier misdeed from his account by balancing it out.

78. Bache, p. 113

From the perspective of the beyond, it is relatively easy to accept even the prospect of a painful coming karmic event, as it still seems rather far away – something like our next week's visit to the dentist's. Thus it is rather easy to decide about one's coming fate. And we will use up some of our "bonus points" of good karma from previous lives, too, to avoid having only to suffer one heavy stroke of fate after the other. Because we have the freedom to choose, we can even choose – despite the many things we still have to balance out in our karmic account – to enjoy this time as a relatively peaceful and pleasurable life. Though our guides may point out the possible waste of an opportunity, but it will be allowed to us "on demand".[79] But at that point we are fully conscious of the fact that all the minus points in our account must be balanced out sooner or later, for "no one can escape what he is due to experience for his unrighteous acts"[80]

"The human soul," says Rudolf Steiner, organizes in the beyond "together with those other humans in karmic relationship and with the beings of the upper hierarchies his coming life in respect to karma."[81] Some leave the details of what will meet them to those higher beings that will later initiate the karmic events, while others want to plan them down to the smallest detail themselves. And, as Pythagoras said, as a rule the more advanced souls will plan their future lives themselves, the somewhat less advanced will decide themselves some parts and leave other parts open,

79. Reincarnation therapy is in disagreement with Shankara and Vyasa, who think that karmic balancing has to occur in the next following life. But then our free will would be limited.

80. Harder, p. 223

81. quoted in Hummel,p. 92

whereas the little advanced will leave everything up to their karma guides (called *lipika* by Indians [from Sanskrit: scribe or clerk]).

But everyone has given their approval to their coming fate before they enter into a new human life. That is required by the law of free will. Because nothing should happen to them on earth against their will. In other words, the fate that we experience on earth is not only determined as karmic reaction from our earlier lives, but is in addition a result of a decision on the basis of personal insight and individual free will.

These details are new within research on karma and cast a new light on the law of karma itself. Because at the point of entering upon a new life on earth we have not only understood the law of karma and accepted its positive value, but we have accepted its practical application, even in the strictest sense, to our own lives. Thus every life on earth is prescribed – either directly or indirectly – and approved ahead of time by us personally. Because we connect with every stroke of fate some concrete aim, a step on the path leading us to "becoming love".

Michael Newton describes the case of a soul that asks to be able to experience in its coming life being raped as a woman, "in order to understand...and estimate the destruction that it had as a man caused the (raped) girl".[82] And we remember the Germanic warrior who had burnt a child with fire set to a hut and wished in the beyond to be killed by burning in its next life (Case 1).

But only the spiritually very advanced will have this higher insight that the actual fundamental reason for painful events is the necessary experience of the opposite of all-

82. Newton I, p. 51

harmony and all-love. So only very few are able to recognize this "inner will", as Aurobindo would call it. For the others the validity of the law of karma is a plausible – and therefore sufficient – reason to subject themselves to its sway.

We can also make an agreement with members of our group to learn something together in a new incarnation, i.e. to support and aid each other as friends, spouses, partners, family members or relatives. Most of these agreements are made with the object of learning in the school of life; only seldom are they aimed at pure mutual enjoyment.

For certain reasons it may be advisable for our teachers, leaders or consultants to choose souls from another group for our mission, if there are no suitable souls in our own group. Because it is the new learning mission together with the need for karmic balancing that have priority, other components such as land of birth, parents, birth-date and length of life being of secondary importance.

Elisabeth Kübler-Ross can still remember asking a friend in the beyond – before her present birth – why he had decided to take birth and die of hunger as a child in Africa. He answered, "Such a life would expand my compassion", explaining that he had lacked compassion for others in his previous life.[83] But not all that which is hard to bear in our lives and which we have chosen explicitly for our new life is necessarily connected to our earlier lives and the karma resulting from them. Edgar Cayce[84] is right to point out

83. Kübler-Ross I, p. 20
84. Cerminara quotes a Cayce-Reading in which a man with muscular dystrophy was described who did not chose this illness on karmic grounds but because he "wanted to acquire the virtues of peacefulness and steadiness by means of this condition". (Cerminara, 250)

that one can also establish a fate for oneself that is karma-free (cf. above: The 23 Kinds of Karma, 22. Karma-free karma). I am therefore free to decide, e.g., to help others by becoming a mongoloid child. I can also wish to be born with a crippled foot, so that I no longer can run after material things as in my last life, but can use this life for intellectual or spiritual purposes. But here at any rate I am the architect of my own world. In this special case causality is established voluntarily and under my own direction. So not every life must have its roots in karma – though almost all do - but it must have its roots in causality planned beforehand.

If a woman experienced in her past life many problems on account of her beauty, she may wish to be unattractive or she may say, "No, I want to be just as beautiful again and prove that I am strong enough to withstand all temptations. For I have just learned here how to act properly and would like to test my ability to put it into practice." Of course this will be allowed – if she sticks to this decision. For her own good, though, her guides will surely try to convince her to "take it easy" and try to gain more experience before she faces such strong temptation again.

So we take a look at our karma account to see what we have to balance out, but we also take advantage of our bonus points. Another example: wealth. If we want, we can be born rich or become rich. But perhaps we know the danger of money already from an earlier life of our own or from the descriptions of other group members. By having wealth one can easily become entangled in possessions, so that one is not the possessor but the possessed. And one can easily become guilty of hard-hearted actions, which then have to be balanced out again. In contrast to the dreams and wishes of most people on earth, lives in wealth are therefore generally avoided, unless one wants to test his ability to avoid falling into the pit of hard-heartedness.

The period in the beyond before entering into a new incarnation is used for intensive preparation. The coming situations are practiced in role-play, and there may be training for the coming occupation, as we saw in case 2, where the soul of the Russian trader acquired the necessary knowledge in herbs needed for its coming earth life. This explains, for instance, the phenomenon of child prodigies: either they have brought their knowledge with them from other lives or they receive training in the beyond before beginning their next life.

We also choose whether to be born as a man or a woman, depending on what we are planning to balance or learn on earth. As pure spirit we are actually neuter. But once having entered into duality and having accepted a soul in order to experience the opposite of the All-Oneness, we have to choose one of the two sexes for each incarnation. The choice of sex is also up to us and can change from incarnation to incarnation.

But usually an extended program with one sex or the other is chosen. If I need to learn to manage power, then I will usually choose several masculine lives. If, on the contrary, the theme is motherhood, I will need a number of female lives. Because here, too, there is much to learn: I can be the mother of a handicapped child in order to learn to be very loving and kind to my child. I may also learn to be the mother of many children or to be a single mother living in great poverty. And I can also learn a lot if my children die one after the other. But generally these different experiences are spread over several lives. Because each life is filled with many different learning tasks.

The karma planners and consultants make sure, though, that no one takes on more than he can manage in his new earthly life. Therefore Elisabeth Kübler-Ross says with conviction in her speeches, "One never gets more than what one can bear." That means that each burden on earth, even if it seems too heavy from the earthly perspective, is exactly proportioned for the soul that has to carry it and, no matter how big it appears, it never is too much for one to manage. Therefore it should be borne courageously until the end. Anyone who is hesitant and gives up hope, perhaps even taking his own life or becoming a hermit, has no gain, none at all, but only the certain fate of having at some time in the future to repeat the same program from the beginning.

And we can remember that every life must be optimal for us, having been carefully planned down to the smallest detail and the learning tasks having been set – or at least accepted – by ourselves. Whoever hesitates or is disheartened while facing a new life has twice as hard a time going through. The person that approaches the task courageously and unhesitatingly will master it more surely. Therefore: take courage, "become friends" with your karma and enjoy your life! Because we are also the creator of our own lives, and –by living in agreement with our inner commandment of love – we can make them happy ones! If our karma meets us in the form of war, illness, accident or in any other form, we should not despair but take it "by the horns" and do the best we can to master it.

We can also choose our parents. But our karma consultant may say that the chosen parents are completely inadequate for the planned program, e.g. that the father is much too gentle to beat the child as the karmic program requires. Or, if the soul will not change its mind, then it is arranged that the father separates from the mother, who then marries someone else to fill the role of a merciless drillmaster.

Youths up to puberty cannot create karma and then only to a limited amount until they are bodily mature. But even as babies they may be recipients or balancers of karma: if, e.g., I once abused a child, then I must be abused as a child.

If the plan "in which the amount of the punishment and its length has been established" and approved, then the soul "approaches the punishment voluntarily".[85] Plotinus had thus already recognized in Roman time that karma is already prepared, understood and accepted in the beyond, being "the most wonderful of all rooms for sense perception"[86]. This is true knowledge that was not regained until we learned to do empirical research on the beyond by means of Regression Therapy.

Wars and catastrophes are also planned in detail beforehand for karmic reasons because they offer a good opportunity to provide many people at the same time with the possibility of karmic learning and balancing. The karma of each of those involved is already specifically built in to all wars or natural catastrophes, and they have also been approved or tacitly accepted (i.e. by the karma recipient's having left the details up to his councilors).

And a special boon is given to those ready to reincarnate but just waiting for the proper and fitting karmic slot to be prepared for them. They are allowed to forget what they have experienced in earlier lives, in order to make their

85. Harder, p. 223
86. Harder, p. 211

passage through the new life as unbiased as possible. Because if one could remember what had taken place in one's former life or in the beyond, one might suffer from self-accusations – e.g. as a previous murderer – and not be able to carry out one's plan in an open manner. Or it might be too easy if one knew the whole life plan including time of death or the agreements already made in the beyond. Therefore, as the great researcher of death Elisabeth Kübler-Ross says, the angel of forgetfulness comes and erases all our memory of the past before we enter into the womb of our new mother.[87]

The hour of death is surely planned already. But eventual changes are already foreseen in the plan, e.g.: "If you finish your 'curriculum' (learning plan) early, you can leave this school of life earlier." Or: "If you have attained all the knowledge you intended to by the time you are seventy, you can still remain as long as you want in order to learn some more or just to enjoy your life a little longer."

But most souls do not want to stay a second longer than necessary on earth. And when I asked Elisabeth Kübler-Ross why it is then that we come to earth in the first place, if everything in the beyond is so nice, she said, "The earth is a school of life. We have to learn in this unpleasant physical zone what we couldn't learn on the other side. Because on the other side we experience unconditional love. How could we learn to love if everything is so rosy? Here we have to learn to get along with nasty and cruel people, with disgusting politics [etc.] in order to experience how to manage negativity. As long as we have not learned this

---

87. Kübler-Ross I, p. 25, „If we already knew what would happen, we would not grow or learn anything new. We would be a population of dummies."

lesson, we have to return again and again to this world, until we have learned it. Therefore we have to return many, many, many times until we have finally attained a level of consciousness where we can understand that we are not separated from each other, but are always and at every moment in union with each other. When we really know that and can live accordingly, then we can die, never to return to earth again."[88]

When and how can karma come to an end?

In general we can say that karma is only over when it has been balanced, i.e. equalized. Because that is the law. But karma, if it is negative, is always a sign that one has broken the laws of love. The purpose of karma – except for original karma – is to help us learn to love. If, however, we could manage to eliminate what we have accumulated out of callousness (lovelessness) before the inevitable law of karma strikes, karmic reactions would no longer be necessary. Karma as a medium for learning love would be superfluous if we could reach the goal of living in pure love without its help.

Thus when we live – to use the expression of my dear teacher Elisabeth Kübler-Ross – in "*unconditional love*", i.e. if we in our thought, speech and actions have become totally loving, we will have attained the goal of our earthly lives and will not need to return to the earth again. As soon as we attain this goal, any possible remnants in our karma-book will be erased, for they would have become irrelevant at that time. Why should a car be sent to pick up someone who has already returned home?

88. Kübler-Ross I, p. 10

With love self-awareness, too, is linked. Because I have to come to the point where I am aware that the whole of creation is composed of love and that I am a part of this love. As soon as I am aware of this fact, I will also act accordingly. Dick Sutphen's central idea is, "Wisdom dissolves karma." I would state this even more exactly: Karma is dissolved through wisdom and love.

But how can I reach this goal, so that my remaining karma can be eliminated? As we heard at the beginning of this book, great Indian masters claim that one need only turn to them in full trust and love and follow their rules in order to attain freedom from karma. And thousands of people take this path. But I think that just as we have to die alone, we also have to go this way alone.

Certainly it is easier to die when we are accompanied by someone. And a spiritual master can accompany someone on the last stretch before the final goal. And perhaps there is loving energy that the master can transmit to the disciple, so that his frequency may suddenly be raised and the goal of his becoming love himself may be reached more quickly. Millions of people who have experienced *darshan*, being in the presence of the master and feeling his aura and his love, have sensed a sudden raising of their own love vibrations, putting them into a more ecstatic state. *Darshan* can change a person completely and set him on the path of love forever.

Rationally oriented people cannot understand how so many persons can make themselves dependent on a guru or master. But the latter do not want them to be dependent – truly wise teachers of love tell their disciples to become their own gurus. But what drives them again and again to

89. Sutphen II, p. 110

their revered masters is the wish to taste love from such a wonderful source.

If we have become total love, we cannot act otherwise as according to the laws of love. We can no longer break them. Because on the long path through our many incarnations we have learned that any deviation from the path will draw corrective measures in its wake, with which – as negative karma – we have become sufficiently acquainted. We have been led to unconditional love by experience. Now we can love unconditionally all humans, animals, plants, indeed the whole of creation. If we carry this love in us, it is impossible for us to deviate from the proper path of love. All of our thoughts, words and acts are in agreement with divine all-love, and we follow the laws of all-harmony. We have become completely and consciously united with creation and its laws.

And now some readers might say, "I can never reach that point, as long as I am on earth!" But in the divine creation this has already been arranged for. Just as in our final exams in school not everyone was able to attain the highest marks in all subjects, also in our last earthly incarnation we do not have to have already reached the state of pure love. Because that may only be possible for a few of us. But after passing successfully our final examination on earth we will have the opportunity in the beyond to learn the last steps to love perfection. After that, if we are willing, we can return to the unity of all-harmony and all-love, in order to live in the fullness of joy and love – now bringing all our newly gained experience of the opposite of all-harmony and all-love to bear on this life. And through our remembrance of this opposite we will be able to appreciate the glories of the divine all-harmony and all-love all the more.

But perhaps one or the other of us (as, according to Tibetan belief, also Buddha did on account of his great love for the living beings) will decide to renounce the joys of immediate return to the Oneness, wishing to be of service to those souls who are still in the process of becoming total love.

But what do I have to do to pass my "examination" perhaps already in this life? Very simple! I have to become in my thinking, speaking and acting complete love. If I attain this, then all further karma will be erased from my account. And it is helpful to know the spiritual laws. Because if one understands intellectually the principles on which these laws are based, it is easier to understand love and the divine creative will dwelling in these laws and thus to put them into practice.[90] If one lives responsibly and lovingly on the path of divine law, one will be free from all karma.

Every book that awakens and supports one's love should be seen as welcome present. Every person I meet who is living in love is a benediction on my way to perfection in love. And even every animal demonstrating unconditional surrender and love to me can become a teacher in love. I should transmit vibrations of love with a wide-open heart vibrating in harmony with all other loving frequencies. In this way I can recognize the love that is in abundance everywhere, though sometimes in a hidden form. For, whatever I send, I will also receive.

And then I should learn to feel the love felt for me by those invisible persons accompanying me. If we are able to make contact with them, we can learn so much from their

---

90. I would recommend in this connection the book by Kurt Tepperwein, *Die Geistigen Gesetze (The Spiritual Laws).*

love about love itself. Because they, if they are already somewhat advanced, think, speak and act out of pure love. They can be good examples and companions on the way to love.

Some rules of thumb for spiritual life are:

- Do no willful harm to anyone. Follow the path of righteousness (dharma) and love.
- Don't let your ego get you to take advantage of someone else.
- Never think negatively. If it happens nonetheless, follow it up with three positive thoughts.
- Forgive everyone who has done anything wrong to you or caused you suffering. Ask everyone you have done wrong to or caused suffering – whether in words or in thoughts – to forgive you. In this way you can possibly prevent or reduce a karmic reaction. Begin right away to forgive others. You can gain strength for this by prayers. If you ask, you will be given help from above.

It is no coincidence that humans have been graced at the end of the 20th century with Regression Therapy as an instrument in attaining love. Because Regression Therapy opens up the possibility of dissolving the still existent karmic remnants of those gigantic purification and balancing events of the 20th century (and not only for those directly concerned!). Because in this type of therapy the client gains either from his guides or other beings in the beyond, from his Higher Self or from his own higher consciousness on the Mountain of Revelation: He learns about higher love and understands karmic entanglements, how they arise and how they can be dissolved. He offers the cup of love, of forgiveness and of dissolution of suffering and guilt to all those persons entangled with him in earlier lives and in his present life. And he forgives them all and himself in love. This love, which he experiences in Regression Therapy, will keep on vibrating in him for a long time, perhaps even putting him in a state of love-vibration, thus allowing him to follow consciously from then on the path of dharma and love and to complete in love up to the last breath his last life on earth.

Quotations and Aphorisms

One becomes what one thinks. That is the whole secret.

(Upanishads)

Don't do that which you wish others not to do to you.

(Confucius)

I myself was already born as a boy and a girl and was already a plant, bird and dumb fish in the waters of the sea.

(Empedocles)

Everyone's life is the result of his former life. One's former mistakes are evident now as suffering and pain, whereas the earlier good deeds show their benedictions.

(Gautama Buddha)

The Ruler and Master of this world has established the fortune and misfortune of all beings as well as their happiness and sorrow according to their previous lives.

(Mahabharata)

Just as the calf finds its mother among a thousand cows, the previous deeds follow on the heels of their perpetrators.

(Mahabharata)

The fate of someone cannot be separated from his past and future: everyone has determined his present fate in an earlier life and is now preparing his future fate.

(Plotinus)

I died as a stone and became a plant. I died as a plant and advanced to become an animal, finally I became a human. I will even surpass the angels to become what no man has seen. And then I will be nothingness.

(Dschaladin Rumi, founder of Sufism)

Pleasure and pain were not given us by others;
That others give us these is madness.
Everyone enjoys in his time
What he committed in the past.
Suffer yourself, oh body, what you have done. (from an Indian poem)
Why shouldn't I come again as often as I am sent to get new knowledge, new abilities?

(Gotthold Ephrahim Lessing)

Whoever doesn't attain perfection here will perhaps attain it there in the beyond, or he will have to take another turn on earth.

(Novalis)

In comparison to reincarnation and karma all other opinions seem small and negligible.

(Richard Wagner)

Whatever one was not able to do in one existence, one will do in another. So no one can avoid the law of progress. Everyone is rewarded according to his real value.

(Allan Kardec)

The law of karma is the basic law of the universe, which binds the effect to the cause in the physical, mental and spiritual world.

(Helena P. Blavatsky)

Karma is the eternal assertion of human freedom. Our thoughts, our deeds and the threads of the net which we through around ourselves.

(Swami Vivekananda)

We all return again. All life only has meaning on the basis of this certainty. And it is completely irrelevant if in a later life we remember our earlier ones. Because the individual person and his memory and satisfaction are not important. Only the great impulse to perfection matters, the impulse to purification advancing in every incarnation.

(Gustav Mahler)

All battles and competitions in animal and plant life and everywhere else, all social conflicts and wars are only the expression of the eternal effort to return to that state of equality.

(Swami Vivekananda)

We are slaves of the past but the lords of the future.

(Rudolf Steiner)

As a rule a human does better the second time than at his first attempt.

(Rudolf Steiner)

Just as an avalanche falling down a mountainside does not indicate a moral but rather a natural process, in the same way suffering breaking upon a person does not indicate a moral but just a causal punishment.

(Paul Brunton)

We choose our joys and pains long before we experience them.

(Khalil Gibran)

If the bad things that we suffer now are the result of the sins committed in our past lives, we can endure them with humility and with the hope that our future lives will be less painful if we strive in our present one for virtue.

(William Somerset Maugham)

Our life is not only of our own making. For the most part it stems from hidden sources. Even complexes can begin a century or more before birth. There is something like karma. (C.G. Jung in a letter to Eleanor Bertine, 1946)

If a person is constantly aware of the law of karma that good deeds reap good results and bad deeds bad ones, he will shudder on thinking of carrying out bad deeds and be happy when carrying out good ones

(Munishri Nyayavijayaji)

Man is responsible for purifying the sparks in the things and beings he meets in daily life and for raising them to ever higher levels, to ever higher births, from mineral, from plant to animal, from animal to man, until the holy spark can return to its origin.

(Martin Buber)

Karma is a wonder of precision whose purpose lies in changing your direction.

(Sai Baba)

Reincarnation and karma exist so that everyone has the chance to learn from his own mistakes.

(Sai Baba)

Consider always that everything that happens to you is the best that could happen and that your task is to find out why this is so.

(Sai Baba)

Whenever we break the law of karma we have to pay back.

(Daskalos)

Since we daily create the blueprints for tomorrow, awareness of the karmic law provides the insight we need to bring our lives into harmony with that law.

(Hazel Denning)

We have not yet learned to love and serve our fellowman. Until we do, we will continue to suffer all manner of diseases and psychological pain.

(Hazel Denning)

Everyone must eat the fruits of his own fields.

(Liz Green)

A universal grasp and understanding of the nature of the law of tikune (karmic law) could change the entire world. If people really accepted this principle, they would be far less inclined to exploit their fellows on this planet, and the idea of "love thy neighbour" would be regarded as a practical rule of thumb rather than a remote ideal.

(Rabbi Philip Berg)

The karmic system is a far better source of justice than any legal system that has ever been devised by humanity.

(Bruce Goldberg)

It is not the purpose of karma to reward or to punish. Its purpose is to educate the subconscious, and to purify it.

(Bruce Goldberg)

No one has an experience that he is not pre-destined for.

(Inayat Khan)

An appreciation of our patterns takes the sting from our pain and makes of life an interesting adventure.

(Ernest Pecci)

It is not fate that makes our lives difficult but the decisions we made earlier - whose consequences we feel now as karma.

(Ingrid Vallières)

The law of karma was not invented to punish us but to sharpen our senses and our awareness of our deeds.

(Ingrid Vallières)

You should love your fate because it is your best chance to make progress. The whole of life is a learning process directed by fate.

(Stefan von Jankovich)

Whoever bases his fortune on the misfortune of others will find in his next life his own misfortune.

(Kurt Tepperwein)

Everyone is the creator, carrier and master of his own fate. Fate is the sum of our decisions. Thus there is neither unearned fortune nor unearned misfortune but only cause and effect. It is the most just of all possible laws. It says, "Everyone reaps what he sows."

(Kurt Tepperwein)

The law of karma demands of man that he takes responsibility for himself and his life. It makes sure that he will be confronted with that which he himself has created until he has been able to eliminate it and therefore become free.

(Kurt Tepperwein)

It is not possible to carry out something and escape its results. No one can do injustice without suffering injustice.

(Kurt Tepperwein)

Our fate is nothing other than the sum of our right and wrong decisions. Every apparent injustice is a higher justice.

(Kurt Tepperwein)

Everyone must be reborn again and again until he experiences the results of all the causes initiated by him, thus fulfilling the law.

(Tepperwein)

The law of karma binds the ignorant but makes the wise free.

(Kurt Tepperwein)

Whoever is consciously one with the will of creation will be totally free of karma. He will bring about no new cause for new karma.

(Kurt Tepperwein)

Accept karma as the basis of your life philosophy. In that way you will accept full responsibility.

(Dick Sutphen)

All of your positive and loving thoughts and deeds contribute to erasing your accumulated bad karma.

(Dick Sutphen)

Regression Therapy is really a wonderful way of processing symptoms, but it can be much more. It supports us on the way to salvation and complete healing, for it meets the highest demands even in a religious sense.

(Ruediger Dahlke)

People who actively seek to work out their karma appear to receive protection from divine forces. ... It does not release them from their karmic debts, but it strengthen them and enables them to move forward in a more positive and directed manner.

(Richard Webster)

One of the most powerful ways of releasing karma is to forgive others and yourself.

(Richard Webster)

Man is punished by his sins, not for them. Karma neither rewards nor punishes; it only restores lost harmony.

(Christmas Humphreys)

Regression Therapy is too valuable only to be reserved for the ill ones.

(Erving Polster)

In that group of persons which you despise, hate, humiliate or exploit the most you will be reborn.

(Jan Erik Sigdell)

The Law of Karma says: no debt in the universe goes unpaid.

(Deepak Chopra)

Whether you like it or not, everything that is happening at this moment is a result of choices you have made in the past.

(Deepak Chopra)

The karmic law makes everyone responsible for his actions. If every mean person would know that for all his deeds he will be once responsible for, we could envisage a wonderful world ahead of us.

(Elisabeth Kübler-Ross)

Everyone reaps what he sows. Karma is therefore the most just of all laws.

We are the planters. Our crop depends on how well we prepare the field and on which seeds we sow.

If we distance ourselves from love, we will be removed from love. If we open ourselves to love, we will be blessed with more love.

If deep in your heart you hate a people, a religion, a race, you have earned with that a guarantee that you will voluntarily be born among them.

Everything that I do to someone else I have thus done to myself, for I am the other one. Because we are all one.

The law of karma is a merciful gift of God. It allows me to take care of my salvation myself – at whichever speed I choose.

Everything that we take from others will at some time be taken from us. Therefore honesty is the best preparation for our later life.

There is no place for chance in God's wonderfully conceived creation.

The grosser our offense against love, the more callously we will be treated ourselves.

He who knows does not lament, for he knows why everything is as it is.

Illness is an expression of karmic disharmonies that is crying for harmonization.

Fate is the mirror of my soul. It reveals my past to me.

Karma is the product of my own independence. Therefore I cannot give anyone else the blame.

The law of karma is not to be equated with fatalism. On the contrary, it orders us to take measures, in order to meet a preferable fate in the future.

Karma is not the enemy of mankind but its best friend. Karma is not a barrier for our union with God but its accelerator.

Karma is not mechanism for punishment but a system of education – or better: a system orienting us towards true becoming love.

The law of karma is practical education by example. It pressures us to look at our insufficiencies. And these are: too little love.

Karma is a motor for our development. Without it we would develop very little or even stand still.

We should be thankful for karma because it only wants the best for us. It wants to force us to look at our mistakes, so that we can become perfect in love and thus create the preconditions for our reunion with all-love.

Death is only the end of our school day, returning home, relaxing and resting, reunion with family members and friends, doing our homework and preparation for the next school day.

The law of gravity and the law of karma have one thing in common: the deeper one falls, the greater the damage.

Regression Therapy makes it possible to learn about karma and thus to reconcile ourselves to it.

Karmic partnerships are the preferred polishing sandpaper, where the souls can polish each other down to the point where they become perfectly shining loving souls.

To forgive ourselves and others in love allows us to end our karma early.

Painful karma is nothing else than deeds born out of

callousness that have not yet been balanced by love.

Whoever knows correctly the cause of his fate will no longer suffer because of it, for he knows why everything is as it is. It is ignorance that makes us suffer.

We inherit ourselves from life to life. Whoever would like to have a good inheritance should manage his life so that his inheritance is a pleasant one.

Everything you send out comes back to you. Send out love. And you will see what happens.

The law of karma is the instrument that teaches us to love. Only by the lovelessness with which we treat others and which accordingly we have to experience in our next life do we gradually recognize the value of love. Karma is thus the most valuable instrument for becoming love.

Self-knowledge and self-realization as an all-loving person are the preconditions for realization of the divine.

Just as we only learn the value of water when we are in the desert, we only learn the value of love in the wastelands of life. And karma sends us again and again into the wasteland of life, until we really have learned the value of love, yes, until we have really become love in our thoughts, speech and acts.

Through lovelessness we experience the value of love.

Karma dissolves itself through wisdom and love.

That in which we have made our mistakes in love requires our balancing. God's law wants it like that. And there is nothing more to add.

Bibliography

General Introduction to Karma and Reincarnation

Atkinson, William Walker: *The Law of Karma*, 1908

Bache, Christopher M.: *Lifecycles: Reincarnation and the Web of Life*, New York 1990

Brunton, Paul: *Essays on the Quest*, London 1984

Brunton, Paul: *What is Karma?*, New York 1998

Cerminara, Gina: *Many Mansions*, New York 1967,

Cranston, Sylvia and Williams, Carey: *Reincarnation*, New York 1984

Currie, Jan: *You Cannot Die*, New York 1978

Friedli, Richard: *Zwischen Himmel und Hölle – Die Reinkarnation*, Freiburg, Schweiz, 1986

Head, Joseph and Cranston S.L.: *Reincarnation – The Phoenix Fire Mystery*, New York 1979

Hummel, Reinhard: *Reinkarnation – Weltbilder des Reinkarnationsglaubens und das Christentum*, Stuttgart, 1988

MacGregor, Geddes: *Reincarnation in Christianity*, Wheaton Ill., 1978

Mumford, Jonn: *Karma Manual*, St. Paul 1999

Schmidt-Leukel, Perry (Hrsg.): *Die Idee der Reinkarnation in Ost und West*, München 1996

Tendam, Hans: *Exploring Reincarnation*, London 1990

Tepperwein, Kurt: *Schicksal und Bestimmung*, Güllesheim 2001

Zürrer, Ronald: *Reinkarnation – Die umfassende Wissenschaft der Seelenwanderung*, Zürich 1989

Zürrer, Ronald: Weg nach Innen, Neuhausen, CH 1995

Western Descriptions of Karma and Reincarnation

Breaux, Charles: *The Way of Karma*, York Beach, Maine 1993

Cayce, Edgar I: *Edgar Cayce on Reincarnation*, New York 1967

Cayce, Edgar II: *Reincarnation – Claiming Your Past, Creating Your Future*, San Francisco 1988

Cayce, Hugh Lynn: *Edgar Cayce's Story of Karma*, New York 1972

Flemming, Beatrice: *Das theosophische Weltbild*, München 1976

Forêt, Pierre de: *Die Geburt der Seele*, Güllesheim 1999

Hanson, Virginia (Hrsg.): quotations from the German editon *Karma – Wie unser Tun zum Schicksal wird*, Bern 1992 (*Karma: Rhythmic Return to Harmony*, Wheaton, Ill. 1990)

Harder, Richard (Hrsg.): *Plotins Schriften*, herein specially the chapter *Probleme der Seele*, Hamburg 1962

Kafka, G. und Eibel, H.: *Der Ausklang der antiken Philosophie und das Erwachen einer neuen Zeit*, Band 9, München 1928

Kübler-Ross, Elisabeth, I: *Warum wir hier sind*, Güllesheim 1999

Mac Gregor, Geddes: *Reincarnation in Christianity*, Wheaton 1978

Kugler, Walter: *Rudolf Steiner und die Anthroposophie*, Köln 1991

Markides, Kyriakos C. I: *The Magus of Strovolos*, New York 1985

Markides, Kyriakos C. II: *Homage to the Sun*, New York 1987

Markides, Kyriakos C. III: *Fire in the Heart*, New York 1990

Sachau, Rüdiger: *Westliche Reinkarnationsvorstellungen*, Gütersloh 1996

Steiner, Rudolf: *Die Offenbarungen des Karma*, Dornach 1985

Steiner, Rudolf: *Wiederverkörperung und Karma*, Dornach 1994

Zander, Helmuth: *Geschichte der Seelenwanderung in Europa*, Darmstadt 1999

Evidence for Reincarnation

Banerjee. H. N.: *Americans Who Have Been Reincarnated*, New York 1980

Hardo, Trutz: *Wiedergeburt – die Beweise*, München 1998

Hardo, Trutz: *Children Who Have Lived Before*, Suffron Waldon, UK 2001

Harrison, Peter and Mary: *Life Before Birth*, London 1983

Leek, Sybil: *Reincarnation – The Second Chance*, New York 1974

Lenz, Frederick: *Lifetimes – True Accounts of Reincarnation*, New York 1979

Mackenzie, Vicki: *Reincarnartion –. The Spanish boy whose destiny was to be a Tibetan Lama*, London 1988

Rogo, D. Scott: *The Search for Yesterday*, Englewood Cliff,NJ 1985

Stevenson, Ian: *Twenty Cases Suggestive of Reincarnation*, Charlottesville 1974

Stevenson, Ian: *Children Who Remember Previous Lifes*, Charlottesville 1987

Stevenson, Ian: *Reincarnation and Biology – a Contribution to the Etiology of Birthmarks and Birth Defects*, Westport,

Connecticut 1997

Stevenson, Ian: *Where Reincarnation and Biology Intersect,* Westport, Connecticut 1997

Books on Reincarnation and Reincarnation Therapy

Andrews, Ted: *How To Uncover Your Past Lives,* St. Paul 1996

Binder, Bettye B. : *Past Life Regression Guidebook,* Culver Cita, CA 1992

Bolduc, Henry Leo: *The Journey Within,* Independence, VA 1988

Bolduc, Henry Leo: *Life Patterns, Independence,* VA 1994

Bowman, Carol: *Children's Past Lifes,* New York 1997

Brennan, J.H.: *Discover Your Past Lives,* New York 1994

Brennan, J.H.: *The Reincarnation Workbook, – A Complete Course in Recalling Past Lives,* Irthlingborough, Northhamptonshire 1989

Denning, Hazel M.: *Life Without Guilt,* St. Paul, 1998

Finkelstein, Adrian: *Your Past Lives And The Healing Process,* Malibu 1996

Goldberg, Bruce: *Past Lives, Future Lives,* New York 1982

Goldberg, Bruce: *The Search for Grace,* St. Paul 1997

Goldberg, Bruce: *Soul Healing,* St. Paul 1997

Hardo, Trutz: *Das große Handbuch der Reinkarnation, Heilung durch*

Rückführung, München 1998

Hardo, Trutz: *Entdecke deine früheren Leben,* München 1997

Linn, Denise: *Past Lives – Present Dreams,* New York 1994

Lukas, Winafred Blake: *Regression Therapy – A Handbook for Professionals,* Volume I and II, Crest Park, 1993

Moody, Raymond A. & Perry, Paul: *Coming Back – A Psychiatrist Explores Past-Life Journeys,* New Yoork 1991

Newton, Michael, I: *Journeys of Souls,* St. Paul, 1995

Newton, Michael, II: *Destiny of Souls*, St. Paul 2000

Norman, Ruth & Spaegel, Charles: *The Principles and Practice of Past Life Therapy*, El Cajon, CA,1984

Oppenheim, Garrett: *Who Were You Before You Were You?* New York1990

Rossetti, Francesca: *Psycho Regression*, York Beach, Maine1992

Sagan, Samuel: *Regression – Past-Life Therapy for Here and Now Freedom*, Sydney 1996

Schlotterbeck, Karl: *Living Your Past Lives*, New York 1987

Sigdell, Jan Erik: *Rückführungen in frühere Leben*, Bern 1998

Sutphen, Dick I: *Enlightenment Transcripts*, Malibu, CA, 1986

Sutphen, Dick II: *Lighting The Light Within*, Malibu, CA, 1987

Sutphen, Dick III: *Predestined Love*, New York 1988

Sutphen, Dick IV: *Reinventing Yourself*, Malibu, Ca, 1993

Vallières, Ingrid: *Past Life Recovery*, Ashgrove Press1997

Wagner McClain, Florence: *A Practical Guide to Past Life Regression*, St. Paul

Webster, Richard: *Past-Life Memories*, St. Paul, 2001

Weiss, Brian: *Many Lives, Many Masters*, New York 1988

Weiss, Brian: *Through Time into Healing*, New York1993

Weiss, Brian: *Only Love Is Real*, New York 1996

Whitton, Joel L. und Fisher, Joe: *Life Between Life*, New York 1986

Williston, Glen & Johnstone, Judith: *Discovering Your Past Lives*, Guildford, Surrey 1988

Woolger, Roger J.: *Other Lives, Other Selves*, New York 1988

Reincarnation and Karma in Buddhism and Jainism

Dalai Lama: *The Four Noble Truths*, London 1997

Dhammananda, K. Sri: *What Buddhists Believe*, Kuala Lumpur 1987

Munishri Nyayavijayaji: *Jaina – Philosophy and Religion*, Delhi 2000

Nemichandra Siddhanta Chakravarti, Shri: *The Sacred Books of the Jainas*, Vol. VI, Lucknow 1927

Oldenberg, Hermann: *The Doctrine of the Upanisads and Early Buddhism*, Delhi 1991

Saalfrank, Eva: *Der Buddha und das Rad der Lehre*, Ulm 1997

Snelling, John: *Buddhismus – Ein Handbuch für den westlichen Leser*, München 1991

Sogyal Rimpoche: *The Tibetan Book of Living and Dying*, San Francisco

Tenzin Gyatshol: *The Opening of the Wisdom-Eye*, Wheaton, Ill. 1981

Reincarnation and Karma in India

Aurobindo, Ghosh, Sri, I: *Der Integrale Yoga*, Hamburg 1957

Aurobindo, Ghosh, Sri, II: *Rebirth and Karma*, Wilmont, WI 1991

Aurobindo, Ghosh, Sri: *Life Divine*, Pondicherry 1970

Bhagavadgita, Ashtavakragita – Indiens heilige Gesänge, München 1992

Darshan Singh: *The Secret of Secrets*, Dehli 1991

Kirpal Singh: *The Wheel of Life*, Delhi 1965

Doniger O'Flaherty, Wendy: *Karma and Rebirth in Classical Indian Tradition*, Delhi 1999

Halbfass, Wilhelm: *Karma und Wiedergeburt im indischen Denken*, Kreuzlingen/CH 2000

Malhotra, Sharan: *Lord Kabir*, Delhi 2000

Osho Rajneesh: *The Zen Manifesto – Freedom From Oneself*, Cologne

Ramakrishna Math: *Sayings of Sri Ramakrishna*, Mylapore, Madras

von Stepski-Doliwa, Stephan, I: *Sai Baba spricht über Psychotherapie*, Grafrath 2000

von Stepski-Doliwa, Stephan, II: *Sai Baba spricht über Beziehungen*, Grafrath 1995

von Stepski-Doliwa, Stephan, III: *Sai Baba spricht über die Welt*, Grafrath 1997

von Stepski-Doliwa, Stephan, IV: *Sai Baba spricht zum Westen*, Grafrath 1994

Swami Rama: *Freedom from the Bondage of Karma*, Honesdale, PA 1977

Zimmer, Heinrich: *Philosophies of India*, New York 1951

Reincarnation and Karma in Judaism

Besserman, Perle: *The Shambhala Guide to Kabbalah and Jewish Mysticism*, Boston 1997

Bischoff, Erich: *Die Elemente der Kabbalah*, Wiesbaden 1990

Berg, Philip: *The Wheel of a Soul*, New York 1988

Gershom, Yonassan: *Beyond the Ashes*, Virginia Beach 199

Gershom, Yonassan: *From Ashes to Healing*, Virginia Beach 1996

Ribner, Melinda: *New Age Judaism*, Deerfield Beach, FL 2000

Scholem, Gerschom: *Kabbalah*, New York 1974

Der Sohar, Das Heilige Buch der Kabbala, München 1998

Winkler, Gershon: *The Soul of Matter*, New York 1992

Other Recommended Reading

Borgia, Anthony: *Life in the World Unseen,* London 1981

Edith Fiore: *The Unquiet Dead,* New York 1988

Hardo, Trutz: *Molar – ein Siebenfarbroman,* Neuwied 1985

Hardo, Trutz: *Lilia – ein Siebenfarbroman,* Neuwied 1995

Hardo, Trutz: *Jedem das Seine – ein Siebenfarbroman,* Güllesheim 1997

Hardo, Trutz: *Maria – ein Siebenfarbroman,* Güllesheim 2002

Hardo, Trutz: *Der Blinde Dichter – Ein Reinkarnationsroman,* Berlin 2001

Kübler-Ross, Elisabeth, II: *On Life After Death,* Berkeley 1991

Schuré, Eduard: *Die Großen Eingeweihten,* Bern 1965

Tepperwein, Kurt: *Die geistigen Gesetze,* München 1992

Tepperwein, Kurt: *Wissen, Handeln, Sein,* Güllesheim 1998

Wickland, Carl: *Thirty Years among the Dead,* Los Angeles 1924

e-mail: tom.hockemeyer@debitel.net or
mail@trutzhardo.de

Homesites: www.trutzhardo.com and www.trutz-hardo.de